KU-470-734

HEALING
WITH
MAGNETIC
THERAPY

Dr. Sarah Brewer

Health Journalist of the Year 2002

D. JAY LTD

113 POPE STREET, BIRMINGHAM, B1 3AG

FIRST PUBLISHED BY D. JAY LTD 2002.

Reprinted 2012

© Dr Sarah Brewer 2002

ISBN 0-9540771-0-5

Printed and bound in Great Britain
All rights reserved.

Compilation by Jayne Langley

FOREWORD

by Torben Hersborg

Osteopath Torben Hersborg is a therapist to numerous Olympic athletes, including Modern Pentathletics gold medallist Dr Stephanie Cook. He was born in Denmark and trained at the European School of Osteopathy in Kent, going on to launch his Central London Health Centre in 1993.

Having had the knocks and strains of high level sports participation as an international judo player, he understands how pain can undermine not only professional performance but personal wellbeing.

FORWARD

Pain is an everyday experience for thousands of people throughout the UK. Nearly two thirds of the country's adults have had experience of back pain at some point in their lives, for example. Many others suffer due to sports injuries, arthritis, rheumatism or work-related repetitive strain injury.

Pain has incredibly debilitating consequences. Even performing the simplest day-to-day chores can be extremely arduous, and for some, impossible. Constant physical pain has a detrimental effect on emotional wellbeing too, and many people become depressed as a result. Its effects can extend beyond the individual sufferer, to partner and family as well.

Although no two people are the same, and different treatments suit different individuals, electromagnetic therapy has been successful in alleviating pain for a significant proportion of sufferers.

In this book, Dr Sarah Brewer, whose extensive knowledge of all aspects of natural medicine is impressive, outlines electromagnetic healing's long history of relieving pain of all kinds. In fact, Dr.Brewer herself has successfully used pain relieving patches to treat a jogging-related knee injury.

The therapeutic power of magnets was known to physicians in ancient Greece, Egypt and China more than 4000 years ago. In 1959, surgeons in the US found that amputated amphibian limbs could be regrown when an electromagnetic field was used. More recently, clinicians who have studied the effects of magnetic therapy have estimated that its effectiveness in relieving pain is 85 per cent, considerably higher than many analgesic drugs, and without risk of side effects.

It is to be hoped that this ancient therapy might bring comfort to the legions of pain sufferers throughout the nation.

Contents

What is Magnetic Therapy?

Magnetic therapy is the use of magnets and the electromagnetic fields they produce to help create a beneficial environment that promotes the body's own healing processes.

When therapeutic magnets are applied to the skin, they produce physiological effects in the body as the blood flowing through the magnet's electromagnetic field contains electrically charged substances such as salt ions and the iron-rich, red blood pigment, haemoglobin.

Magnetic therapy *is sometimes also known as magnetotherapy, magnetiotherapy, biomagnetic therapy, or bioelectromagnetic therapy.*

Magnetic therapy is used in over 50 countries world-wide, including Germany, Israel, Russia and Japan, where magnetotherapy has been used and studied for decades.

The North pole of a magnet has the most therapeutic applications, as this complements the negative polarity of the normal, healthy body and promotes natural healing processes. Traditionally, the north pole of a magnet is used to relieve and calm 'hot' pain due to inflammation and infection, while the south pole which has a more stimulatory effect, may be used to relieve cold, aching types of pain such as that associated with poor circulation.

Clinicians who have studied the effects of magnetic therapy have estimated that its effectiveness in relieving pain is 85 percent, considerably higher than for many analgesic drugs, and without the risk of side effects. Relief is usually rapid, with muscle pains for example, often diminishing within 30 minutes.

The electromagnetic fields used in magnetic therapy may be generated by single or multiple magnets, which may produce a static or a pulsed electromagnetic field. Those most convenient for home use include adhesive magnetic patches, magnetic jewellery (eg necklets, bracelets), wraps and mattress pads.

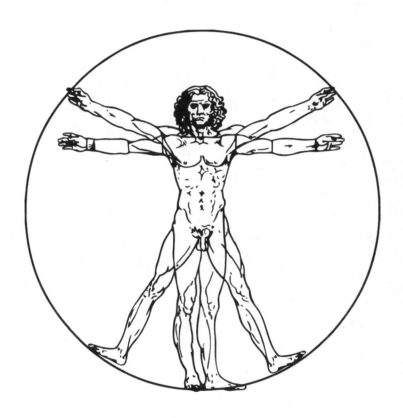

History of magnetic therapy

According to one legend, the phenomenon of magnetism was supposedly discovered, and named after, a Greek shepherd, named Magnes, whose iron staff became strongly attracted to a lodestone rock. Other legends claim that magnetism was first discovered in an ancient part of Europe known as Magnesia.

The therapeutic power of magnets was known to physicians in ancient Greece, Egypt and China over 4000 years ago, who used naturally magnetic rock (known as lodestone or magnetite) to treat a variety of physical and psychological ailments.

Cleopatra (69 - 30 BC) was said to wear a magnet on her forehead to maintain her beauty, and was also said to recommend magnets to treat the gout that was prevalent among her Roman allies. In A.D. 46, the physician Scribonius Largus recommended the use of the electric torpedo fish to cure headaches and gouty arthritis. Ancient Romans also used magnet therapy to treat eye disease, the French physician Marcel used it to treat headaches, and the Islamic physician Avicenna (980 - 1037) to treat depression.

In the 16th Century, the famous Swiss physician and alchemist, Paracelus, was responsible for 'rediscovering' magnetic therapy and used it widely in his practice precipitating a resurgence in its popularity in Europe. He declared that "The magnet is the king of all secrets" and

Cleopatra (69–30 BC)

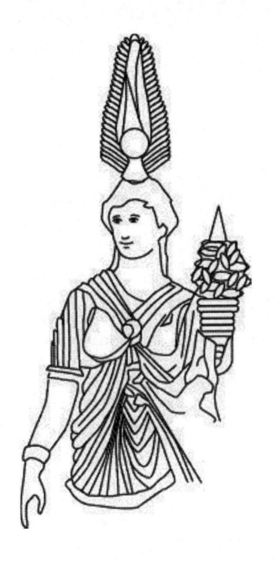

used it to treat a variety of conditions including headache and rheumatic problems. He also recommended drinking a solution made by adding ground lodestone to water.

The 18th Century Viennese physician, Franz Anton Mesmer believed that magnets could enhance a Universal force that permeated the body, which he called 'animal magnetism'.

Today, magnetic therapy is popular in Japan and parts of Europe, but has only recently become widely known in the West.

In 1959, surgeons in the US found that amputated amphibian limbs could be regrown when an electromagnetic field was used.

Animal studies in the early 1970's suggested that it was only the negative pole of a magnet that has beneficial effects on living cells. Around the same time, researchers also discovered that weak electrical currents (which will produce a magnetic field) could enhance the healing of bone fractures, and strong electromagnetic fields are now used by many orthopaedic surgeons to hasten the healing of bone fractures. The reported success rate is over 80%, even in cases of non-union where other procedures had previously failed.

Magnetic therapy is now also used by some doctors to encourage healing of persistent wounds and ulcers, swelling (oedema) and sometimes to treat deep vein thrombosis.

Franz Anton Mesmer

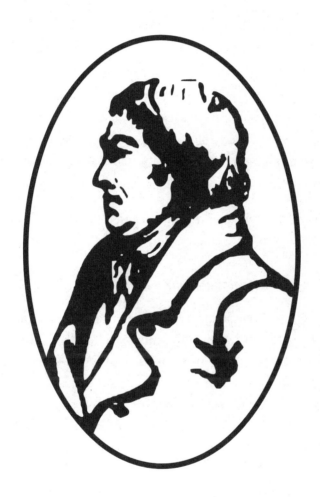

Magnetic resonance imaging (MRI) is also widely used as a diagnostic technique to visualise internal parts of the body, and produces better results, more safely, than using X-rays.

Magnetic Resonance Imaging (MRI)

MRI uses a strong magnetic field to align the molecules in your body. A pulse of radio waves is then passed through you to knock the molecules slightly out of alignment. As the molecules bounce back into place, they give out a weak radio signal which is picked up and interpreted by a computer. This gives an excellent cross-sectional or 3-D image of different parts of your body without any known risks or side effects.

Clinical research into the therapeutic effects of magnetic therapy is also increasing.

What is electromagnetism?

Magnetism is the phenomenon by which certain materials assert an attractive or repulsive influence on other materials. The fact that magnetism exists has been known for thousands of years, since the discovery that natural lodestone (magnetite) could attract or repel iron objects, but the underlying principles of physics that govern magnetism and the related phenomenon of electricity have only been understood within the last hundred years.

The first step in understanding magnetism came when Michael Faraday discovered that a changing magnetic field

A changing magnetic field can produce an electric field

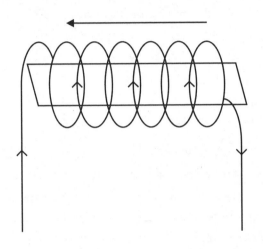

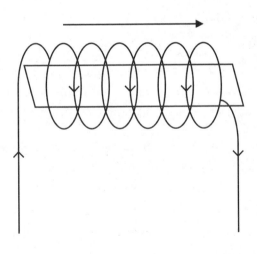

can produce an electric field. For example, if a bar magnet is pushed into a coil of wire, it will produce a measurable electric current flowing through the wire - but only while the magnet is moving. When left stationary inside the coil, it will not produce an electric current, but on being withdrawn again, current will once more flow – the direction of the current will depend on the direction in which the magnet is moving. This is one of the ways in which modern electric power is now generated.

James Clerk Maxwell then deduced that as electricity and magnetism are related, a changing electric field should produce a magnetic field. This can be shown experimentally by passing a wire down through a small hole in a piece of card which has been sprinkled with iron filings. When an electric current flows through the wire, the iron filings on the card will form concentric rings due to the magnetic field generated by the current.

Maxwell also showed that electric and magnetic fields travel together through space as waves of electromagnetic radiation and that their changing fields sustain each other.

Until early in the 20th Century, magnetism and electricity were thought to be two different forces, but in 1905, Einstein's special theory of relativity showed that electricity and magnetism are, in fact, interrelated aspects of a common phenomenon, electromagnetism, although each behave quite differently.

Passing a wire down through a small hole in a piece of
card which has been sprinkled with iron filings

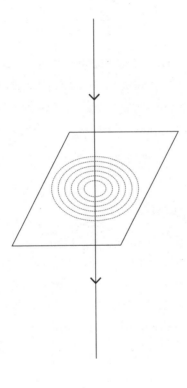

- *Electric forces are produced by electric charges, either at rest or in motion. In contrast, magnetic forces, are produced only by moving charges and act solely on charges in motion.*
- *Electric and magnetic forces are detected in regions called electric and magnetic fields, which can exist in space far from the charge or current that produced them.*
- *Waves of electromagnetic radiation (eg radio waves, microwaves, visible light, X-rays) all travel at the speed of light (around 186,000 miles per second) but differ in the frequency at which their electric and magnetic fields oscillate.*

What is a magnet?

Atoms are made up of a central nucleus, which contains positively charged subatomic particles (protons) and neutral particles (neutrons) surrounded by orbiting negatively charged electrons that are all held together by strong attractive forces. The inside of the atom is positively charged, and the outside negative.

The magnetic properties of materials result from the individual electrons orbiting the atomic nucleus. As it is a moving charge, an electron forms a small current loop which will generate a small magnetic field. Each electron can also be thought of as spinning around an axis which will also produce a small magnetic field.

Atomic Structure

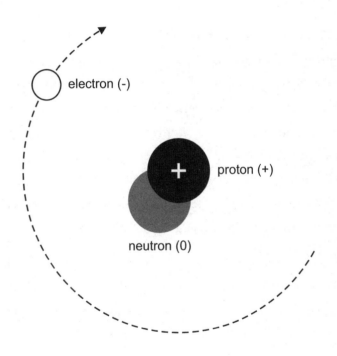

The electrons orbit the nucleus within areas known as shells. If the outer shell contains a full complement of electrons, these form pairs spinning in opposite directions. The magnetic fields they produce cancel each other out, so that the atom to which they belong is electrically stable and unreactive and is not capable of being permanently magnetised.

If electrons are missing from the outer shell, however, the unpaired electrons spin in a haphazard manner which makes the atom reactive, or unstable, and may also allow it to be permanently magnetised. These missing electrons can generate an enormous electromagnetic force – for example, it is calculated that if only one electron is missing out of every billion molecules in two people who each weigh 70 kg and are standing 2 m apart, their bodies would repel each other with a force equivalent to 30,000-tons!

As all substances are made up of atoms containing electrons, all will show some magnetic properties when placed in a magnetic field (eg the pole of a permanent bar magnet), even materials which are not normally thought of as being magnetic. This weak magnetic behaviour, due to induced changes in the orbits of electrons, will only persist for as long as the external field is applied.

Some substances, such as iron, cobalt, nickel, boron and neodymium are more highly attracted towards the pole of a

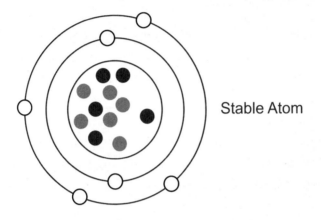

Stable Atom

● protons (+1)
● neutrons (0)
○ electrons (-1)

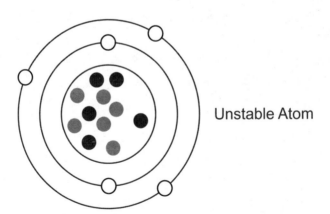

Unstable Atom

permanent bar magnet, however, even a weak one, and are capable of being permanently magnetised as a result of their electronic structure.

In the case of iron, for example, three electrons are missing from its outer shell, so that three unpaired electrons are spinning around the central nucleus. While the piece of iron remains unmagnetised, these unpaired electrons have different directions of spin, and the forces they generate tend to cancel each other out. When the unpaired electrons are influenced by the pole of a permanent magnet, however, they become organised and aligned in the same direction, with the same axes of spin, so that the forces generated by these synchronised electrons add together to create a powerful magnetic force which can persist even when the original external magnetic field that aligned them is taken away.

As the number of iron atoms present increases, so does the number of synchronised electrons and the force they collectively generate. A-large magnet made from a heavy piece of iron will therefore generate a much greater magnetic force than a magnet made from a small piece of iron.

Iron magnets

Lodestone (magnetite) is an iron rich ore (Fe_304) that has become magnetised by lying in the Earth's magnetic field for millions of years. Iron can also be magnetised naturally through being struck by lightening, or subjected to an electric field. In medieval times, blacksmiths noticed that

Iron Atom

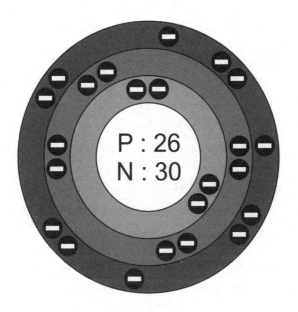

P : 26
N : 30

iron bars could be magnetised if they were heated and then aligned in a north-south direction and beaten with a hammer as they cooled.

In the 1700s, carbon steel was found to retain its magnetism better than plain iron, and in the 1930s, magnets containing iron mixed with aluminium, nickel and cobalt were developed. It was only in the last 20 years that rare earth magnets were developed from metallic elements in the rare earth group of the periodic table of elements.

Rare earth magnets

The modern, therapeutic magnetic patch is made from an alloy of iron, neodymium, and boron. These magnets are made by applying great heat and pressure to the powdered metals and are considerably lighter and more powerful than traditional iron or steel magnets. They are therefore much smaller in size, and can be worn more discreetly (eg applied as a patch) than the traditional magnets that were strapped to the body with belts and bands.

Magnetic patches can be placed directly over a painful site, over acupuncture points, or on various sites of the head.

Measuring magnetic force

The strength of the magnetic field a magnet can produce is measured in modern units known as teslas, after the late scientist, Nikola Tesla (1856-1943). An older measure is also in use, known as the gauss. One tesla is equivalent to 10,000 gauss.

Nikola Tesla (1856–1943)

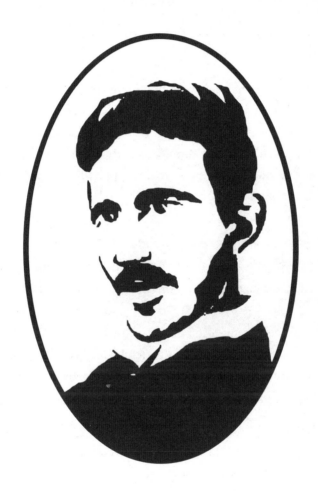

Magnets used in healing usually have field strengths ranging from 0.02 to 0.2 tesla – this is the same as 20 to 200 milliteslas (mT) or 200 to 2000 gauss.

A magnetic field of one gauss is about twice the magnetic field at the earth's surface.

Refrigerator magnets have a strength of 80 to100 gauss, while the medical diagnostic technique of Magnetic Resonance Imaging is done in a field of 10,000 gauss. According to the World Health Organisation, there are no known adverse effects to human health from exposure to static magnetic fields of up to 20,000 gauss.

Low gauss magnets *have a strength of:* **300 to 700 g**
Medium gauss magnets *have a strength of:* **800 to 2500 g**
High gauss magnets *have a strength of greater than* **2500 g**

A high field strength is not necessarily more effective than a low field strength, but as a general rule, look for magnets with a gauss strength of 500 gauss or greater as strengths below this do not seem to be as effective.

Different strengths are used for different applications, and the rare earth magnets used in therapeutic patches produce a field strength of 2000 gauss.

MRI Scanner

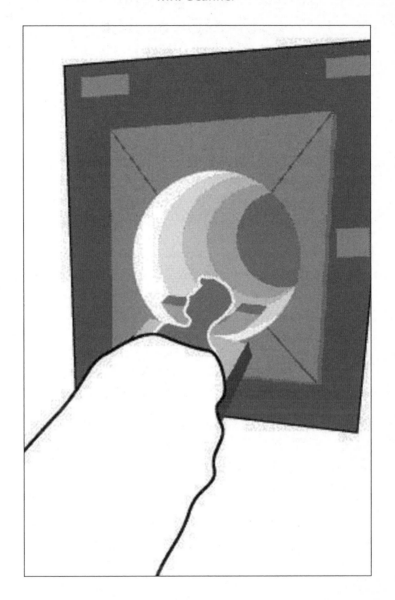

How the body generates an electromagnetic field

All living tissues generate their own delicate electromagnetic fields, which are influenced by a number of external electromagnetic phenomena including the Earth's own magnetic field.

Within the body, it is the flow of electrically charged ions in and out of cells, and the transmission of electric impulses through cell membranes, that are responsible for creating the body's own small but measurable magnetic field.

All your cells are bathed in a fluid containing a variety of dissolved chemicals and salts. Once dissolved, these separate into particles known as ions that carry an electric charge. For example, sodium chloride - common table salt - dissolves to form two types of particle:

- sodium ions that carry a positive electric charge ($Na+$)
- chloride ions that carry a negative electric charge (Cl^-)

Potassium ions are also important for helping to generate electric currents across cell membranes in the body and, like sodium, potassium ions carry a single positive electric charge ($K+$).

Potassium ions are found mainly inside cells, while sodium ions are found mainly outside cells.

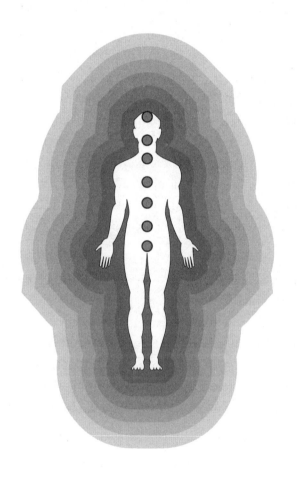

	Sodium ions (Na+)	Potassium ions (K+)
Amount found inside cells	9%	90%
Amount found outside cells	91%	10%

Cell membranes

The cell membrane – known as the plasma membrane - is made up of fat and protein molecules. The fat molecules (phospholipids) are shaped rather like clothes pegs, each with a phosphate 'head' attached to two fatty chain 'legs'. Because of the way the different ends of these molecules either attract or repel water, these 'clothes pegs' line up to form a double layer with the heads on the outside, and the legs in the middle (See diagram). Within this fatty bilayer, a number of larger protein molecules are embedded, which extend from one side of the membrane to the other.

The plasma membrane surrounding each cell is remarkable in that it is semipermeable, only allowing certain substances through, while excluding others. It is this selective permeability that allows an electric potential to build up across the cell membrane. The permeability of cell membranes can also vary so that certain substances are only allowed through under certain conditions, for example, if the cell is damaged, or if the electric potential across the membrane changes.

Membrane 'pores'

The permeability of the cell membrane is controlled by embedded proteins that act rather like microscopic pores through which ions are allowed to flow into, or out of the

The Cell Membrane

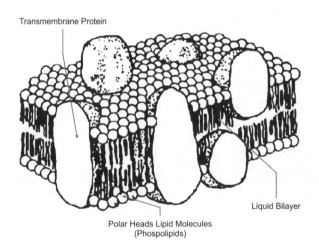

Transmembrane Protein

Liquid Bilayer

Polar Heads Lipid Molecules
(Phospolipids)

cell. Some pores are continuously open, while others are 'gated' and can be either open or closed. Those that are gated may be opened depending on the strength of the electric potential across the cell membrane (voltage gated) or may need a hormone or other chemical trigger to open them.

Pores also vary in their complexity. Some act like simple channels through which molecules diffuse, while others act as carriers that bind molecules, and then change shape, flipping inside-out to bring the bound substances from one side of the cell membrane to the other.

Cell membrane channels *that only transport one substance are known as* uniports.

Channels *that transport* more *than one substance are known as* symports

Channels *that* swap *one substance for another are known as* antiports.

When carrier proteins move substances across the cell membrane in the direction of their chemical or electrical gradient, no energy input is needed and this process is known as 'facilitated diffusion'. Some of the most important membrane pores actively move substances across the cell membrane against a concentration gradient, however, so they become more concentrated on one side than on the other. This is known as 'active transport' and the membrane proteins involved are known as pumps. One of the most

Diagram of a Symporter

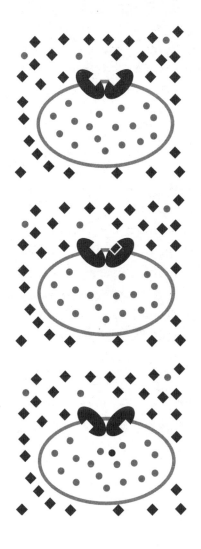

important membrane channels is the sodium-potassium pump, which is classed as a voltage-gated, antiport.

Sodium-potassium pump

The sodium-potassium pump forces sodium out of your cells by swapping it for potassium which is forced inside your cells. This is why sodium is the main positively charged ion found outside cells (in the extracellular fluid) while potassium is the main positively charged ion found in the fluid inside your cells (intracellular fluid).

The sodium-potassium pump transports three positively charged sodium ions out of a cell for every two positively charged potassium ions it transports in. It is therefore an electrogenic (electricity-producing) pump as it produces a net movement of positive charge out of each cell. This net loss of positive charge from cells is also reinforced by a special potassium 'leak' channel, which allows some potassium ions to move out of the cell against their concentration gradient before being pumped back in again by the sodium-potassium pump. This tendency of potassium to leak out of cells is not matched by movements of sodium as the membrane is generally much less permeable to sodium than to potassium.

As a result of these ion changes, the inside of the cell is negatively charged compared with the outside of the cell, and there is a potential difference across the membrane of most – if not all living cells. The electrical charge across cell

Sodium Potassium Pump

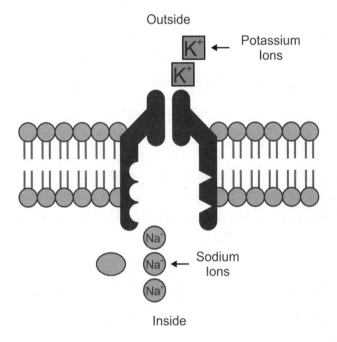

membranes, known as the membrane potential, is given a negative sign (-) by convention, and varies from - 9mV to -100 mV in different tissues. It averages around -70 millivolts (mV) in human nerve cells.

Concentration of various ion inside and outside a spinal nerve

ION	Concentration inside cell	Concentration outside cell
Sodium (Na+)	15 mmol/l	150 mmol/l
Potassium (K+)	150 mmol/l	5.5 mmol/l
Chloride (Cl-)	9 mmol/l	125 mmol/l
Resting membrane potential = - 70 mV		

The movement of positive and negatively charged ions in and out of cells means that every cell acts like a mini battery to produce a minute electric current, and the movement of electrically charged ions in and out of cells is the main source of the body's electrical field. As moving electric charges generate a magnetic field, it is also one of the main sources of the body's magnetic field.

Interestingly, the active transport of sodium and potassium ions in and out of cells is one of the main energy-using metabolic processes occurring within the body. It is estimated to account for 33% of energy (in the form of glucose fuel) used by cells overall, and 70% of energy used by nerve cells alone.

Sodium Potassium Pump

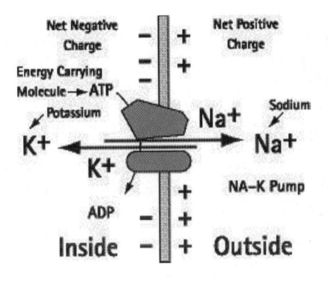

The membrane potential is important for:

- passing electrical messages along nerve fibres
- helping cells to communicate with one another
- helping muscle cells contract – including those in the heart.

When a cell capable of electric activity (eg a nerve cell) is activated, ions quickly flow in opposite directions so that the inside of the cell becomes positive and the outside of the cell negative. This condition – known as depolarisation – only lasts for a short time before the cell returns to its original resting state with the inside of the cell negatively charged compared with the outside. This is accompanied by the flow of a substantial electric current through the active cell membrane. While human cells only generate small bioelectric potentials measured in millivolts, specialised electric cells in the electric organ of some fish can generate voltages as large as 1000 volts which they use to stun or even kill their prey.

Because moving electric charges produce a magnetic field, the flow of ions in and out of every cell in your body contributes to your own magnetic field. As the human body conducts electricity, and is surrounded by a north-south magnetic field from the Earth, we will also generate tiny currents of electricity as we move through this field, which will also contribute to our individual electromagnetic field.

A Nerve Cell

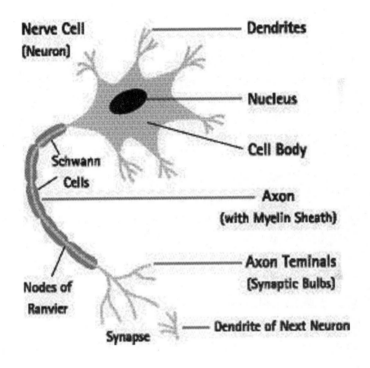

Nerve Cell (Neuron)

Dendrites

Nucleus

Cell Body

Axon (with Myelin Sheath)

Schwann Cells

Axon Teminals (Synaptic Bulbs)

Nodes of Ranvier

Dendrite of Next Neuron

Synapse

Magnetic properties of living tissues

In 1954, Linus Pauling discovered that the iron in the red blood pigment, haemoglobin, is important for cell metabolism and is attracted to a magnetic field along with five other electrolytic salts. Iron makes up around 4% of the haemoglobin molecule, and as iron is so readily magnetised, red blood cells will interact with the beneficial magnetic field produced by a therapeutic magnet brought close to the skin, before travelling around the body and taking some of the benefits of the applied electromagnetic field with it.

Researchers have now also identified areas where magnetite exists within the human brain. They have found minute particles of magnetite (Fe3O4) ranging in size from 50 to 600 nm across, which are present in large numbers - up to 100 million particles per gram of tissue in human brain, and even higher amounts in the membranes covering the brain (pia and dura mater). They seem to be organised in groups of 50 to 100 particles that act as tiny, biological bar magnets. Although the researchers estimate that less than 1 in a 1000 human brain cells contain magnetite, this still represents a large number given that we are each born with over 200 billion brain cells - the same order of magnitude as there are stars in the Milky Way!

The presence of magnetite means that cells can detect much smaller electromagnetic fields than would otherwise be possible, as magnetite allows them to interact over a

Linus Pauling

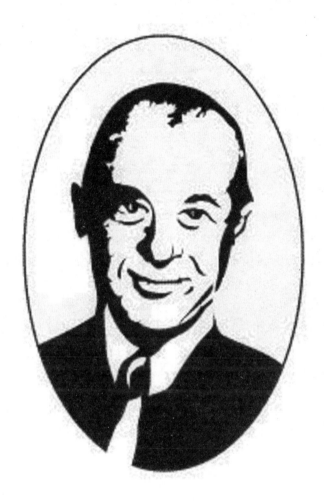

million times more strongly with external magnetic fields than if they did not contain magnetite. Bacteria that contain magnetite crystals are known to use it to orient themselves to the Earth's geomagnetic field, for example, so that they can find the bottom of the ocean. Higher animals such as birds and other vertebrates use magnetite as a navigational aid, although they contain significantly higher concentrations in their cells than have now been detected in human tissues.

The function of magnetite in human brain cells is currently unknown, and it may just be an evolutionary hang-over, or simply a way for cells to store iron. It is more exciting to think that magnetite containing cells may be involved in an as yet unidentified biological receptor system for detecting external low level electromagnetic fields (EMFs), however. They may also play a role in modulating the electrical brain wave activity that is detected in EEG (electroencephalogram recordings) or be involved in detecting the Earth's geomagnetic field, or the Schumann resonances (see page 48) that seem to have a vital stimulatory effect on body cells, healing and growth. Another possibility is that the movement of magnetite embedded within cell membranes might cause cell membrane pores to open or close, to affect the amount of certain substances that can enter or leave cells.

Magnetite in brain cells may also be linked with the production of our sleep-wake biorhythm cycles as magnetic fields seem to affect the amount of melatonin (the body's

EEG Recording of Electrical Brain Wave Activity

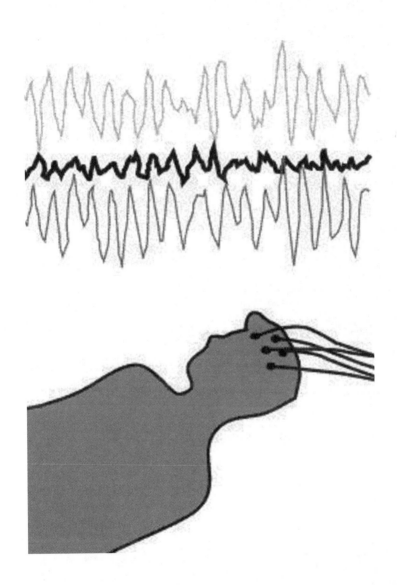

natural sleep hormone) produced in the pineal gland within the brain.

Electrical brain waves recorded by EEG machines show we each produce:

- *Beta waves (14 cycles/sec) associated with feeling energised*
- *Alpha rhythms (8-13 cycle/sec) associated with feeling relaxed, calm and meditative*
- *Theta waves (4-8 cycles/sec) associated with feeling relaxed and experiencing creative bursts of intuitive thought*
- *Delta waves (below 4 cycles/sec) associated with inducing a deep dreamless sleep.*

Electromagnetic fields and illness

Many illnesses affect the electrical functions of cells, and are associated with imbalances in the body's electromagnetic fields, for example:

- damaged cells may leak potassium ions, producing a slow, steady fall in the membrane potential of as much as 50 millivolts
- inflammation alters the transport of ions across cell membranes leading to swelling, redness, increased heat and pain

Electrical Brain Waves

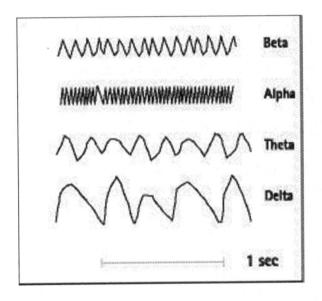

- electrical transmission through nerves is increased when pain is perceived
- when cells die, sudden electric fluxes occur as the cell membrane bursts open, releasing all their intracellular potassium ions in one go
- changes in the composition of blood and in the body's fluid and salt balance will also alter the body's normal electromagnetic field.

Magnetic therapy is believed to access the body's own electric and magnetic fields, and to help realign and correct imbalances to bring relief in a number of common conditions.

Detecting the body's electromagnetic field

Because of the electrical changes occurring within cells, the body generates an electromagnetic field which surrounds everyone with their own individual aura of energy, radiating from the body. The body's magnetic field was first measured by scientists in 1968, and can now be captured on film using techniques such as Kirlian and Aura Energy photography. These techniques suggest that people with a high bioelectromagnetic energy level may have an aura that stretches out a metre or more from their body, while those with a depleted energy level may have an aura that is only a few centimetres wide.

Aura of Energy

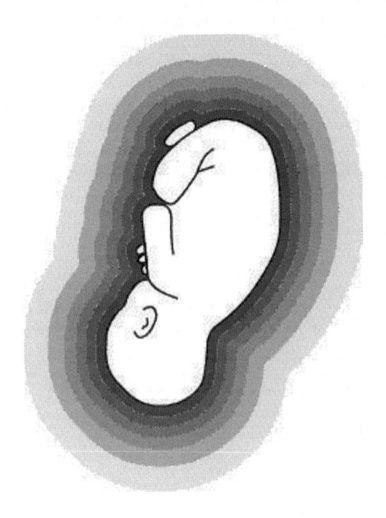

The aura

Some people are particularly sensitive to the body's electromagnetic fields, as are many animals, including sharks who partly locate their prey through detecting their electromagnetic field. Some people say they can sense the aura of others as a vibrational energy while others claim to see them as coloured lights.

You can detect your own aura energy by rubbing your hands together briskly for a minute, then slowly separate your hands and gently pull them apart, regularly pushing them slightly closer together until you can feel the presence of an energy field between your two palms.

The aura is made up of a variety of colours which flow into one another and which change from moment to moment. These can be captured with Aura Energy photography to show how your aura appears at that moment in time. Often, one colour (red, orange, yellow, green, blue, indigo, violet or white) dominates. When you have your aura photographed it shows how your aura is at that particular time, but if you were to have the image taken later the same day, subtle differences would be seen. If taken later in the week, perhaps when you were more stressed, it might be significantly different again.

The human aura is believed to have seven layers that relate to the seven chakras. The inner layer which is closest to the

Aura Energy Photography

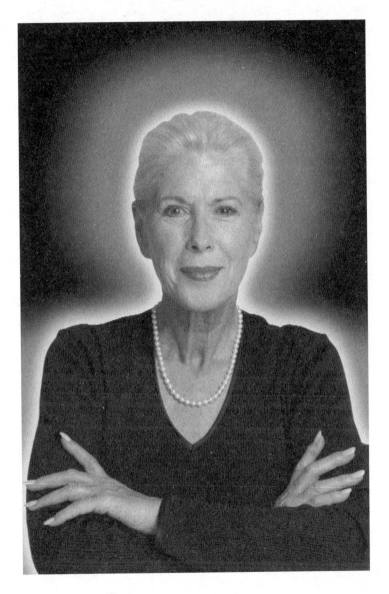

skin relates to health, while the outer layer is the spiritual layer. The Chakras act as gateways between the aura and the body's energy distribution channels. Although this may sound mystical, there is every reason to believe that these ancient beliefs are based on facts which are only now becoming scientifically verified. You can buy a hand-held acupuncture device in most chemists, for example, that can measure electrical resistance across the skin and which can accurately pinpoint acupuncture points as sites where this resistance changes.

Kirlian photography

The quality of the body's electromagnetic field can also be photographed and analysed using Kirlian photography. A part of the body – usually the hands and/or feet – are placed on a photographic plate that emits a high-voltage, high frequency electric signal which can be felt as a slight, buzzing sensation. The way your energy interacts with this frequency is captured on film as an interference pattern. The shape and intensity of the images obtained relate to your electromagnetic aura and can reveal energy imbalances between both sides of the body to diagnose ill health. The energy images are also related to the acupuncture meridians.

Kirlian Photography

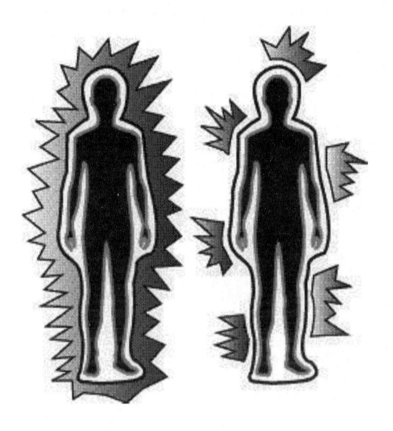

Aura of a
Healthy Body

Aura of an
Unhealthy Body

Factors that can affect the body's electromagnetic field

As we have seen, every living thing generates its own electromagnetic field, which is influenced by our metabolism, state of health, by illness, and by the external electromagnetic fields to which we are exposed.

One of the strongest electromagnetic forces we are subjected to is that of the Earth. When our planet was formed, over 4.4 billion years ago, the slow rotation of the Earth's crust around the molten metal core generated forces of heat and friction which magnetised the iron-rich crust, creating a magnetic field across the globe from the North to South poles. This was estimated to have a strength of 4.0 gauss – more than ten per cent stronger than that which is present today.

The Earth's surface has a natural electromagnetic field of around 7.8-15 cycles per second (Hz, named after discoverer Heinrich Hertz).

The Earth's north pole currently has a negative magnetic polarity, and the south pole is currently positive although these polarities are known to reverse from time to time. So, if you are in the northern hemisphere, you are in the Earth's negative (-) magnetic field, while if you are in the southern hemisphere you are in a magnetic field that is positive (+). In either location the earth's field passes through your body in one direction – the effects of jet lag may partly be due to

Earth's Electromagnetic Field

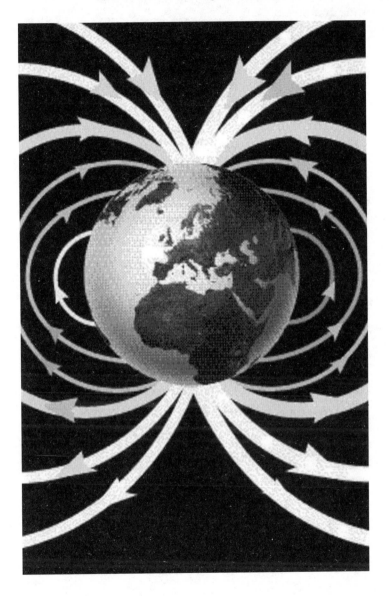

changing magnetic fields on the body, as well as changing time zones.

Our cells' electrical activity has evolved within the Earth's static magnetic field, and it seems to be vital for health and for optimum immunity. We are also subjected to electromagnetic fields generated by thunderstorms in the equatorial zones. These produce natural, low-frequency (7.8Hz) vibrations in the atmosphere – known as Schumann resonances – that seem to have a vital stimulatory effect on our body cells, healing and growth.

NASA have found that animals and humans will not survive in space unless their spacecraft are provided with a magnetic field similar to that of the Earth. This is because the movement of ions and conduction of nerve messages within our cells need the correct electromagnetic environment in which to function properly. If deprived of the Earth's electromagnetic field, severe metabolic disturbances occur including abnormal cell uptake of electrolytes such as calcium, needed for heart muscle. Because cells cannot function properly outside these resonances, they are now incorporated into space craft design so astronaut's are not deprived of their beneficial effects.

Another major electromagnetic force that acts on our cells is that of the sun, especially at times of sunspot activity and solar flares. We are now also surrounded by alternating electro-magnetic fields produced by modern alternating electrical currents that change direction 50 to 60 times per second.

Schumann Frequencies

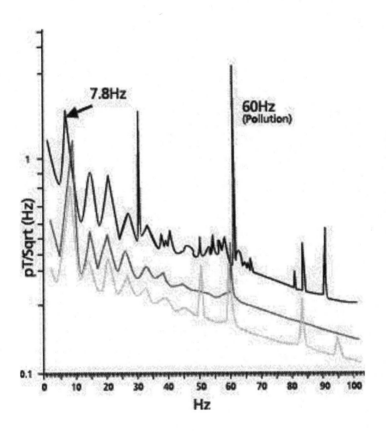

Examples of the variety of factors that can affect our electromagnetic field are shown in the following table.

Factors that can affect the body's electromagnetic field

| External factors | | Internal factors |
Natural	Artificial	
flowing water underground	x-rays, Cobalt-60, radium implants, nuclear reactors	stress
crashing waves on shore	high-tension electric cables, Cellphone transmitter masts, Electrified railway lines, Orbiting satellites	hormone imbalances
thunderstorms	Cordless phones, mobile telephones, answer-machines, fax machines	infection
	Computer screens, laptop computers, computer games,	dietary deficiencies
cosmic rays	Electric sockets, standard lamps, desk lamps, extension cords	excessive alcohol intake
sunspot activity	Television, radios, CD players	drugs
solar flares	Electric fires, hotplates, ovens, microwave ovens, kettles, fridges, freezers, vacuum cleaners, hair dryers, irons, electric blankets and other domestic appliances	
planetary configurations	nuclear fallout	puberty
eclipses	food additives	ovulation
moon phases	irradiated food	pregnancy
x-rays	cooking in aluminium	menopause
gamma rays	sound vibrations	injury
radioactive substances	mercury fillings carbon monoxide Pollution smoking cigarettes	

External magnets placed on or near the body for healing purposes will also have an effect on the body's electromagnetic field.

Each of us has an electromagnetic field radiating
4-6 inches from our body's surface

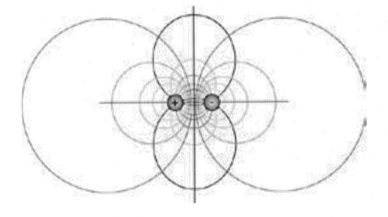

Magnetic field deficiency syndrome

The Earth's magnetic field is slowly decreasing, which may be a precursor to a complete reversal of the Earth's magnetic poles, so that magnetic North will be situated at the geographic South pole rather than the geographic North pole as at present. This shift in polarity has occurred several times in the Earth's history as shown by the way molecules are aligned in ancient, solidified lava flows.

Those working with magnetic therapy believe that good health can only occur when the body is balanced within the earth's magnetic field. This balance is lost when interfered with by the strong electromagnetic fields produced by alternating current in hi-tec items such as power lines, electric blankets and household devices.

We have evolved within a magnetic field of a certain strength, and the fact that this is decreasing means our cells are no longer exposed to magnetic fields of the same strength or quality as that in which they evolved. This, together with prolonged exposure to artificial external magnetic fields – especially those produced by alternating electrical current - is thought to disturb the body's natural resonant frequency leading to cell fatigue and ill health. In 1976, medical researchers in Japan suggested that a disorder known as Magnetic Field Deficiency Syndrome (MFDS) can occur if we are exposed for prolonged periods to electromagnetic fields that are considerably different from

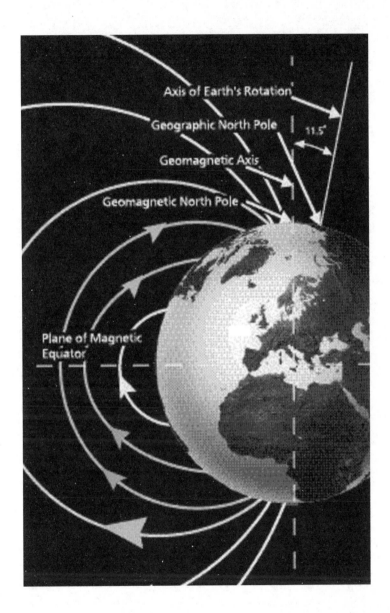

53

our own. Symptoms that are suggested to result from MFDS include:

- muscle stiffness, especially in the back, neck and shoulders
- low back pain
- vague chest pains
- headache
- dizziness
- insomnia
- constipation
- loss of energy
- chronic fatigue.

Correction of magnetic field deficiency syndrome is one of the main aims of magnetic therapy in which direct current magnetic fields or those created by permanent solid-state magnets are used, rather than the alternating current magnetic fields produced by electrical devices. Bioelectro-magnetic therapy is thought to overcome this deficiency syndrome so that these symptoms all improve.

Therapeutic magnetic patches

A variety of magnetic products are now available, including patches, bracelets, pendants, necklaces, clip on magnets, joint wraps, shoe insoles, straps, belts, pillows, car seat covers and even mattresses.

Therapeutic magnetic patches have been developed as an easy, convenient, discreet, natural method of stimulating

A Magnetic Patch

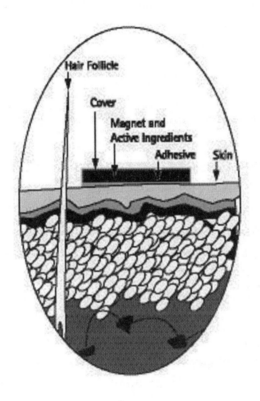

the body's own healing processes to relieve a variety of conditions, including musculoskeletal aches and pains.

Acumed patches

Acumed patches are a patented system that combines magnetic and electrical fields for optimum healing effects. Each patch consists of a hypoallergenic, self-adhesive plaster containing high purity zinc and copper in a magnetic field. The magnetic field is produced by a rare earth magnet (an alloy of neodymium, iron and boron) that provides a field strength of 2000 gauss. The magnet is coated with purified zinc and surrounded with tiny copper spheres, with each element pre-aligned and attached to the self-adhesive, microporous tape to ensure the correct magnetic (negative) pole is in contact with the body. The patch is made from a hypoallergenic, microporous material which allows the skin to breath and is particularly suitable for sensitive skins.

Reproduced by kind permission of Acumed

Each patch works as a mini transmitter, emitting small energy fields which have a soothing effect and stimulate the body's natural pain relief mechanism. Acumed patches generate three different electromagnetic fields:

● magnetic – with the North (negative) pole touching the skin, and the South (positive) pole facing away from the skin

Acumed Patches

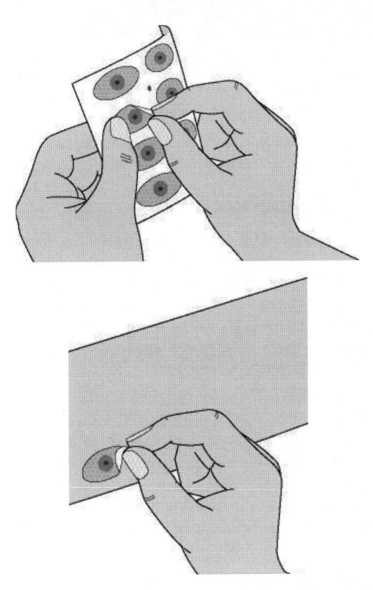

- micro-electric – due to copper and zinc forming a battery bridged by moisture from the skin
- induced electric current – due to the magnetic field acting on the copper microspheres.

These fields interact to produce pulsations of energy that are more effective than using a continuous signal.

Although their exact mechanisms of action is unknown, the electromagnetic energy of magnetic patches is believed to interact with the energy of your own electromagnetic field (aura) to help strengthen it.

Each patch should be applied to clean, dry skin near the site of pain. If positioned over acupuncture points (especially tender tsubos) associated with the painful areas the benefits may be even greater (See page 90). For small areas, or mild to moderate pain, only one patch may prove necessary. If-pain is more extensive or severe, several patches may be used to cover further acupoints as appropriate.

Acumed magnetic patches should be left on the skin, undisturbed, for 5 to 7 days. They can be worn during all normal daily activities, including bathing and showering. After 5-7 days, the Acumed patch(es) should be gently peeled away and discarded. New magnets can be resited as necessary – it is usually beneficial to "rest" for one or two days before re-starting treatment however.

Acupoints

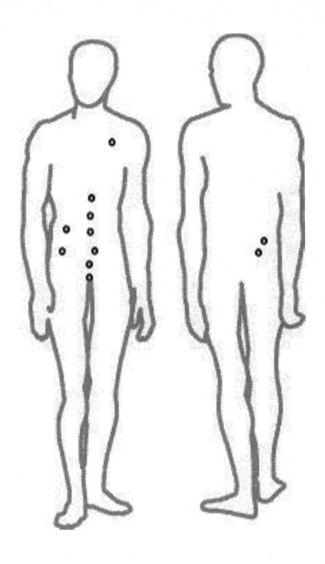

Restoring electro-magnetic balance

Boosting the circulation

Boosting immunity

Regulating enzyme reactions

Regulating the flow of calcium ions

Boosting healing

Producing analgesia

Stimulating production of melatonin

Boosting the Earth's Electromagnetic field

No-one knows exactly how magnetic therapy works, but several interesting theories have been suggested that might explain how it can reduce pain perception and boost healing. Many theories of how magnets work are a variation on what scientists call the Hall Effect. Since our bloodstream is filled with positively and negatively charged ions, stimulating these ions by exposure to a magnetic field generates a certain amount of heat. The heat increases the blood supply to the area where the magnet is located, and with the blood comes extra oxygen and nutrients, as well as a flushing away of toxins.

How does magnetic therapy work?

The electric and magnetic fields produced by the magnetic patches affect the flow of electromagnetic energy in parts of the body. In particular, it frees imbalances and build-ups of electromagnetic energy - often associated with tissue

Flow of electromagnetic energy through the body

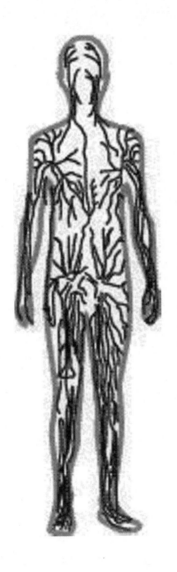

damage and inflammation - that irritate:

- nerves - to cause pain
- muscles - to cause spasm

Magnetic therapy can act on nerve and muscle cells to relieve pain, relax tense muscles, improve the circulation and boost immunity through a number of suggested mechanisms.

Possible mechanism 1: Restoring electro-magnetic balance

Each cell acts as an electro-magnetic unit producing its own magnetic field. During health, cells vibrate with their own characteristic electromagnetic frequency. During disease, a cell's electromagnetic vibration changes. This effect is used to diagnose heart problems for example, using a heart trace (electrocardiogram or ECG). During health, the ECG will show a particular pattern generated by the passage of electrical messages throughout the heart muscle as it alternately beats then rests.

If cells lack oxygen due to reduced blood flow in coronary heart disease, characteristic changes occur in the ECG that help to diagnose the problem quite accurately. In the most simple terms, electromagnetic therapy is believed to restore health by helping cells regain their natural electromagnetic frequency.

Possible mechanism 2: Boosting the circulation

Another theory is that electromagnetic therapy improves blood flow – especially through tiny blood vessels known as capillaries. Red blood cells are coated with a cell membrane

ECG Record of Myocardial Insufficiency

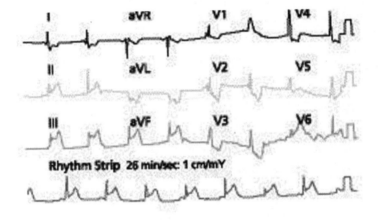

which, like other cells in the body carries a negative (water repelling) charge inside the double layer, but has a variety of positive and negative charges (water attracting) on the surface. These help to repel other red blood cells, and also helps to keep them away from blood vessel walls, so they don't form unwanted blood clots in the circulation. As a result, blood flow is improved – by aligning blood cells in an organised manner which essentially has a blood thinning action. This is similar in principle to the way that magnets applied to water pipes reduce furring up of the pipes, and to the way that magnets applied to fuel pumps reduces fuel consumption.

In the 1950s, it was discovered that when heated, magnetically treated water was less likely to form scale in pipes than unmagnetised water. A water molecule consists of two positively charged hydrogen atoms (H+) and a negatively charged oxygen atom (O2-). Because of the electron configuration of these molecules, the positively charged hydrogen atoms of one molecule tend to attract the negatively charged oxygen atoms of other water molecules. This results in the formation of clusters which can contain anywhere from four to literally hundreds of water molecules. Magnetisation is thought to break up clusters of water molecules that surround lime deposits and other foreign molecules so they remain in the water stream rather than being deposited on pipe walls.

Clusters of 6 water molecules.
Bonds (dark grey lines) connect hydrogren atoms (grey)
to oxygen atoms (black)

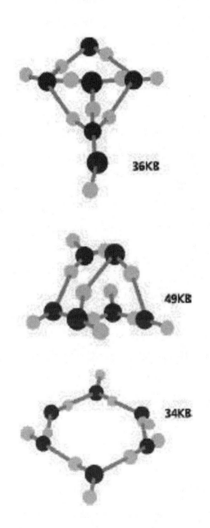

Red blood cells also contain the red blood pigment, haemoglobin, which contains iron – one of the most easily magnetised substances on Earth. In 1954, Linus Pauling received the Nobel Prize in Chemistry partly for discovering the magnetic properties of haemoglobin, each molecule of which contains four atoms of iron.

This means that red blood cells can respond to an electromagnetic field and even become magnetised themselves. Blood also contains copper and dissolved ions (eg sodium, potassium, chloride) that make it a powerful conductor of electric and magnetic currents.

As red blood cells pass through small capillaries in the skin under an applied magnet, they travel through a magnetic field which is believed to produce effects within the haemoglobin molecules that help them carry oxygen to the tissues more effectively. As the charged ions in blood pass through the magnetic field, they inevitably produce a small electric current which will also boost blood flow and strengthen the circulation. In some cases, blood flow is increased by as much as three fold within five minutes. Improved blood flow in turn increases the amount of oxygen, glucose and nutrients available to cells, and flushes away cell toxins, helping to keep tissues healthy and improving healing. Greater oxygenation in tissues also increases resistance to infection.

Possible mechanism 3: Boosting immunity

T-lymphocytes are immune cells that play an important role in the body's immune and inflammatory responses. In order

Diagrammatic representation of a haemoglobin molecule

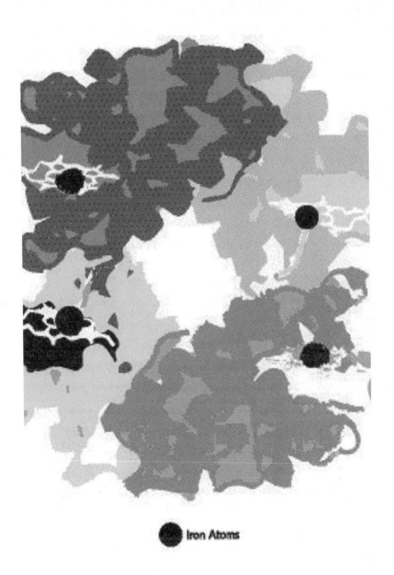

Iron Atoms

to move easily between other cells in the body's tissues, T-cells polarise themselves into tiny magnets (using positively charged calcium ions) so they can move towards an electromagnetic field more easily. These electromagnetic fields are formed in the body around damaged cells, damaged nerves, and electric currents produced by pressure (piezoelectric currents) where bones rub together in arthritic joints. T-lymphocytes therefore accumulate wherever there are unusual electromagnetic fields in the body. Once there, they release powerful chemicals (lymphokines) that attract other immune cells into the area which tends to make the inflammation and pain worse. Magnetic therapy is thought to have a beneficial effect on T-lymphocytes so that they don't over-react and inflammation can resolve more quickly.

Possible mechanism 4: Regulating enzyme reactions

Most metabolic reactions in the body depend on the activity of enzymes – proteins that facilitate the interaction of two or more molecules so that reactions that would otherwise occur at too slow a rate can occur at an accelerated, yet controlled rate. Experiments have shown that exposure to a magnetic field (strengths ranging from 60 gauss to 20,000 gauss for up to 25 hours were used) increased the activity of certain plant enzymes by amounts ranging from 20% to over 90%. Other experiments have found that a magnetic field can also slow the activity of some other enzymes by around 25% with different field strengths having different effects. It is likely that magnetic therapy can produce similar effects on human

Electron micrograph of T-lymphocytes

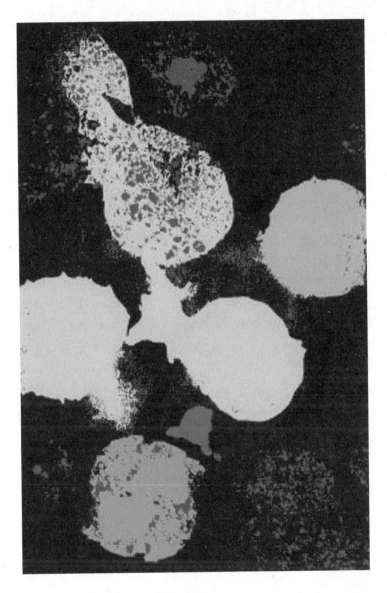

enzymes, by speeding up some reactions (eg to do with healing) and slowing others (eg to do with inflammation).

Possible mechanism 5: Regulating the flow of calcium ions

Magnetic fields affect the chemicals bonds found within calcium bicarbonate molecules, stretching and breaking them so that more is converted into calcium hydroxide (+ carbon dioxide gas which is removed). Over all, this has the effect of improving the alkalinity of extra-cellular fluids. This both increases the amount of oxygen that can be absorbed, and damps down growth of micro-organisms. It also allows mineral ions such as calcium, magnesium, potassium, zinc and chromium to move more freely, ensuring improved cell nutrition and excretion. For example, one magnetic polarity can help calcium move away from painful arthritic joints, and the other magnetic polarity can attract calcium ions towards a broken bone to hasten healing, especially where non-union has previously occurred (See page 134).

Possible mechanism 6: Boosting healing

Magnetic fields seem to stabilise human DNA, to enhance DNA synthesis, and to activate a cell's metabolic processes. These two effects combined seem to boost the healing and repair processes.

Possible mechanism 7: Producing analgesia

Magnets are thought to reduce pain by reducing inflammation (See 3, page 66), by normalising the movement of ions and the flow of electric 'messages' in affected

Human cell with stretched out DNA

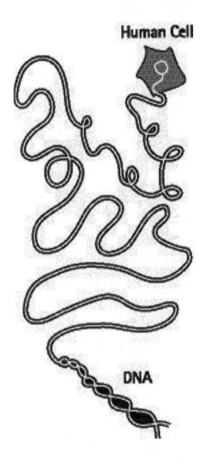

areas, which in turn damps down over-activity of pain receptors, and by stimulating production of the body's natural painkillers, known as endorphins, to damp down pain perception. When levels of endorphins were measured in blood before and after exposure to a static magnet (3950 gauss) for fifteen minutes, endorphin levels were found to increase by 25% one hour afterwards, and by 45% two hours after exposure. Some researchers also believe that the effects of stress hormones cause magnetic imbalances in cells, and that applying the negative pole of a magnet can stabilise or 'repolarise' affected cells which may also reduce pain perception.

Possible mechanism 8: Stimulating production of melatonin

Melatonin is a hormone produced within the pineal gland in the brain. Melatonin has a variety of effects in the body, including helping to regulate the body's biorhythms and sleep-wake cycle and boosting immunity. Exposure to electromagnetic fields emanating from 60 Hz alternating current has been shown to reduce nocturnal melatonin concentrations in electric utility workers, especially if they also worked in low light levels. Another study of 12 men with low back pain also found that exposure to a low-frequency alternating magnetic field for 3 weeks (20 min per day, 5 days per week) either at 10 o'clock in the morning, or at 6 o'clock in the evening experienced a significant reduction in the nocturnal melatonin rise that usually occurs, regardless of the time of exposure although the percentage of

Diagram showing the pineal gland position

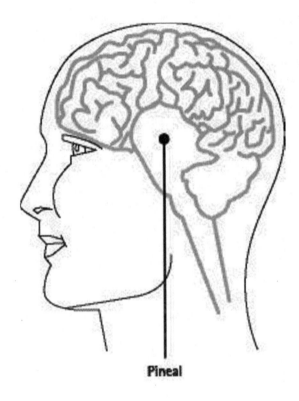

Pineal

inhibition of melatonin secretion varied among individuals. Magnetic therapy may therefore help to offset the effects of exposure to harmful environmental electromagnetic radiation although this is not yet confirmed.

Possible mechanism 9:
Boosting the Earth's Electromagnetic field

The earth's magnetic field has decreased by 50% over the last 500 years. In the last 100 years it has decreased by 5% and is continuing to reduce at the rate of 0.05% per year. Magnetic therapy is believed by some to help boost a cell's degree of exposure to beneficial electromagnetic fields to help offset the fall in background exposure to the Earth's field thereby helping to offset the effects of Magnetic Field Deficiency Syndrome (See page 52).

Earth's Magnetic Field

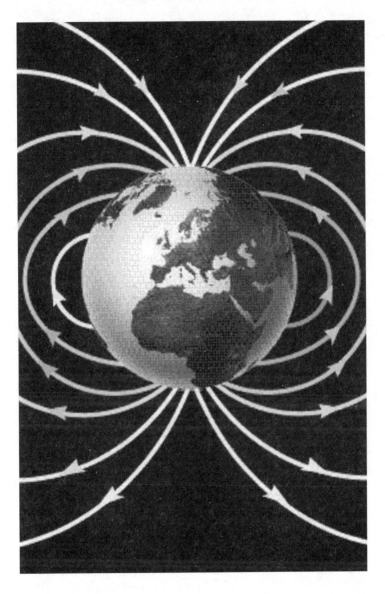

Research findings

Magnetic therapy has long been accepted as a standard medical treatment in Asia, parts of Europe, Australia and is now gaining acceptance in the United States and UK.

The negative field magnets are those most commonly used to alleviate the pain of arthritis and other inflammatory conditions, as well as rashes, burns and general aches.

Musculoskeletal pain

Most of the research into magnetic therapy has been carried out in Japan. Early research findings were so impressive that the Welfare Ministry of Japan granted permission for the manufacture of magnetic pellets to treat rheumatic disorders as long ago as 1972. In one study, magnetic pellets sold over-the-counter included a questionnaire within the pack and, after 11,648 replies were analysed, researchers estimated that the magnetic patches were over 90% effective.

A double-blind study in Japan involving 121 patients with severe, chronic shoulder pain showed that 82% of those treated with high-strength magnets showed significant improvement within 4 days. In those treated with low-strength magnets, there was only a 37% improvement rate. In a similar trial, electromagnetic patches were found to be 80.2% effective in relieving painful, stiff shoulders while non-magnetised placebos were only 6.3% effective.

In another double-blind study involving 222 patients with acute and chronic muscle and joint pain, 90% of patients

Example of a high voltage strength magnet

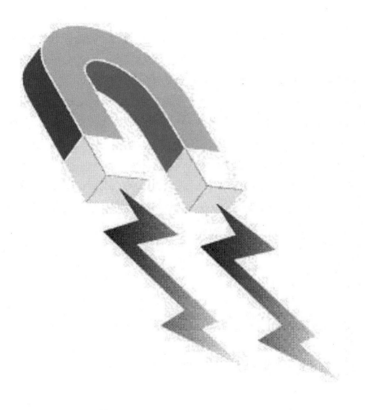

reported significant improvement within five days, compared with only 14% in the placebo group.

Depression

In 1996, a study published in The Lancet found that magnetic therapy could help to treat depression which was failing to respond to antidepressant drugs. Seventeen people with depression were randomised to receive either magnetic treatment, or placebo (dummy magnetic treatment) and were given both treatments at one time or another so they acted as their own controls. After 5 days of daily magnetic therapy to a particular part of the brain, there were significant reductions in depressive symptoms, and in 11 out of the 17 people, pronounced improvement lasted for as long as 2 weeks after the 5 day treatment period. This was suggested as a safe alternative to electroconvulsive therapy that is sometimes resorted to in cases of severe, non-responsive depression.

Diabetic foot pain

A recent study in the American Journal of Pain Management found that magnets significantly decrease foot pain experienced by people with diabetes who have a condition known as peripheral neuropathy. During the four-month study, participants wore pads containing low-intensity magnets continuously on one foot, and non-magnetized pads on the other foot. The pads were switched during the study without them knowing which was active and which was not.

Peripheral neuropathy affects the nerves in your arms, hands, legs, and feet.

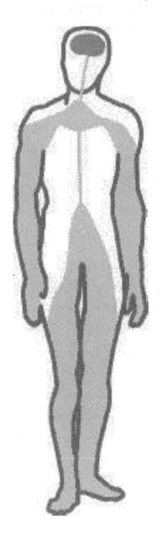

The results showed that the magnetised pads were significantly more effective in reducing diabetic foot pain than the inactive pads. Magnet therapy therefore appears to offer "a real breakthrough" for treating diabetic pain which is often difficult to control.

Menstrual pain
A study in Korea, in which magnet therapy was assessed in 23 student nurses with painful menstrual periods applied therapeutic magnets on the lower abdomen of 11 nurses, and dummy magnets were used with the other 12. Those wearing the real magnets experienced significant pain relief compared with those using placebo.

Post-polio pain
In 1997, a double-blind, placebo controlled study was conducted in the US, investigating the effects of applying a static magnetic field of 300 to 500 Gauss over a pain trigger point in 50 people who had pain following polio infection. Those using active magnets experienced significantly more pain relief than those using dummy magnets. Of the 29 patients who wore active magnets, 76 percent reported a decrease in pain after only 45 minutes. Less than 20 percent of those with the placebos felt an improvement. None of the patients reported any side effects. Most people who have had polio experience chronic pain which is difficult to relieve with drugs. The fact that magnetic therapy can produce rapid relief is an important finding, and the researchers concluded that the "application of a device delivering static

Magnet points for menstrual pain

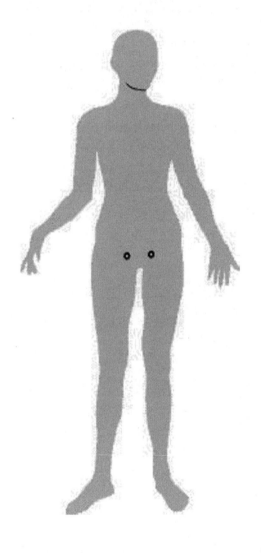

magnetic fields over pain trigger points results in significant and prompt relief of pain." The mechanism by which pain is reduced remains unknown, however.

Chemically induced pain

In 1998, a group of volunteers were reported to have agreed to have a chilli pepper solution injected under their skin. Four neodymium magnets were then applied to the area and found to reduce pain levels significantly!

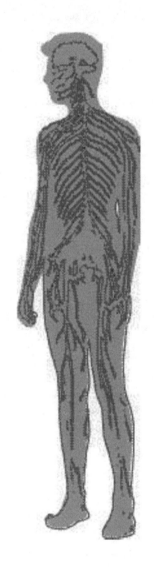

Contraindications

Magnetic therapy should not be used:

- where there is an infection (the therapy may have a beneficial effect on the causative micro-organisms, too)

- in someone who has recently had chicken pox

- on open wounds (except under medical supervision in the case of persistent, non-healing wounds)

- on someone who has recently undergone surgery

- on someone with haemophilia

- on people fitted with a heart pace-maker

- on people undergoing dialysis

- on people using an insulin pump or drug patch

- on people with surgically implanted metal screws

- during pregnancy or while trying to conceive

- on young infants

- if irritation occurs.

The copper component of the magnet may cause slight discoloration on some skin types, but this is harmless and will naturally wear off over a few days.

KEEP AWAY FROM COMPUTER DISCS AND OTHER MAGNETIC MEDIA

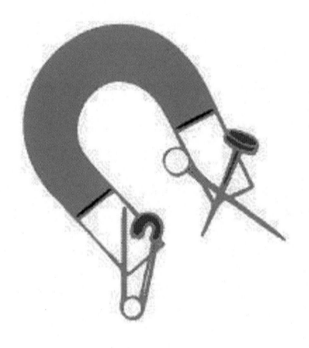

Magnetic therapy, acupuncture and Meridians

Many complementary treatments are based on the theory that the body's energy flows through channels known as meridians, which lie between nerves and muscles. In China, this vital energy is known as Ch'i or Qi (pronounced chee), while in Japan it is known as Ki.

The flow of Qi depends on the balance of two opposing forces: the Yin and the Yang. There are twelve main meridians – six of which are said to have a Yang polarity and are related to hollow organs (eg stomach), and six which are said to have a Yin relating mainly to solid organs (eg liver). Eight further meridians control the other twelve. Along each meridian a number of acupoints have been identified where Ch'i energy is concentrated and can enter or leave the body. Three hundred and sixty five classic acupoints were traditionally sited on the meridians but around 2000 acupoints have now been discovered and are depicted on modern charts. Acupoints have a lower electrical resistance than surrounding areas and can be pinpointed with great accuracy with a simple, hand held device that measures electrical potentials across the skin.

The flow of energy through meridians of different polarity can be compared with the currents that exist in a magnetic field. Some ancient Chinese writings have even suggested that the life force, or qi, was generated by the Earth's magnetic field.

Lung Meridian Acupoints

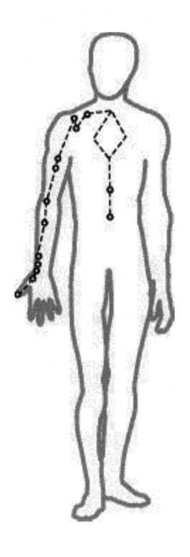

In health, energy flows through the meridians in a balanced way. This balance is easily disrupted through factors such as stress, emotions, poor diet and spiritual neglect however. The symptoms of illness are believed to be caused by blockage of energy flow through these channels. Ill health is thought to be associated with imbalances or blockages in energy flow through the body.

Chakras

The Chakras are seven energy distribution centres that are believed to exist along the midline of the body. Each chakra is associated with a particular colour and is believed to generate or distribute energy to different parts of the body. According to ancient yogic beliefs, meditation, yoga postures and breathing exercises help to encourage a type of energy known as kundalini to move from the lowest to the highest chakra to promote spirituality, higher awareness and divine knowledge. Blockage in an underactive or overactive chakra or along a meridian (energy pathways used in acupuncture) results in pranic depletion or congestion.

Acupoints

Energy flowing through the meridians can be accessed through classic acupuncture points – known as acupoints - on the skin surface. Complementary techniques such as Shiatsu, Acupressure and Acupuncture are designed to stimulate particular acupoints and to allow energy to enter or leave the body at these points, to achieve balance and harmony.

The Seven Chakras

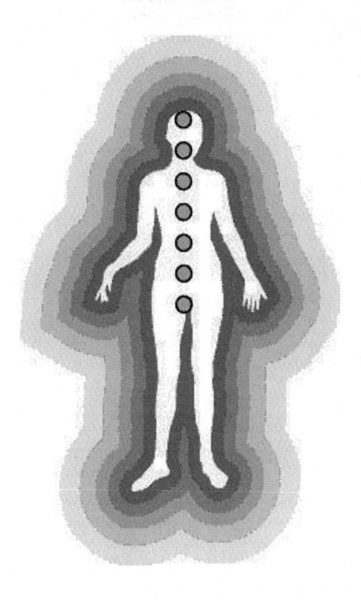

When energy flow becomes abnormal, acupoints on the surrounding skin often become tender and painful to touch. These are known as tsubos. In acupuncture, these points are stimulated with fine needles to generate electrical impulses and restore energy balance.

Magnetic therapy

Magnetic therapy can also be used to access the body's electric and magnetic fields by stimulating acupoints with tiny pulses of electromagnetic energy. This is most easily achieved using rare earth magnets made from an alloy of neodymium, iron and boron. These are coated with purified zinc and surrounded with tiny copper spheres which generate an electric field when connected by sweat on the skin surface. These therapeutic electromagnets are pre-attached to adhesive patches and can be stuck to the skin over particular acupuncture points – or areas of tenderness (tsubos) to relieve pain and stiffness associated with conditions as diverse as arthritis, rheumatic condition, headache, menstrual pain, insomnia and lack of energy. Patches are left undisturbed for 5 to 7 days. Magnetic therapy acts on nerve and muscle cells to relieve pain, relax tense muscles, improve the circulation, boost immunity and energy levels.

How does magnetic therapy differ from acupuncture?

Acupuncture involves stimulating acupoints by inserting and manipulating fine needles to generate electromagnetic impulses. Treatment is usually limited to short sessions spread

Acupoints on the torso

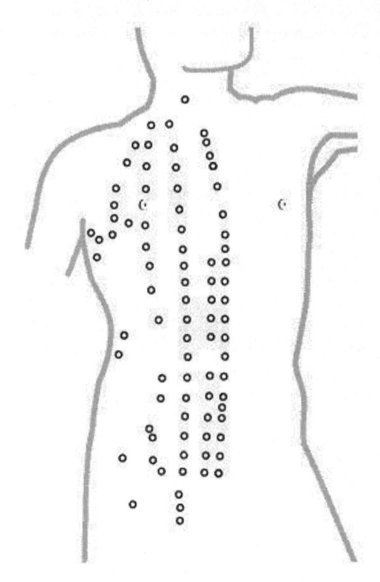

out over a period of time. Magnetic therapy produces a similar effect, but is less invasive. Treatment is also continuous over a period of 5-7 days depending on how long the patches are worn.

How does magnetic therapy differ from T.E.N.S?

Transcutaneous electrical nerve stimulation (T.E.N.S.) delivers strong electro-magnetic pulses to stimulate nerve endings in the skin. This sends pain-blocking signals to the brain and temporarily numbs surrounding tissues. TENS is used to relieve musculoskeletal pain (eg back ache, sports injuries, sciatica, arthritis, tennis elbow) and is also used during childbirth.

In many ways, Acumed patches are a battery-free, smaller version of T.E.N.S. Acumed can be used continuously over 5-7 days however - for as long as the patches are worn - and it emits three different electromagnetic fields. This may be more efficient in stimulating the production of natural pain-relieving substances (endorphins).

T.E.N.S. treatment

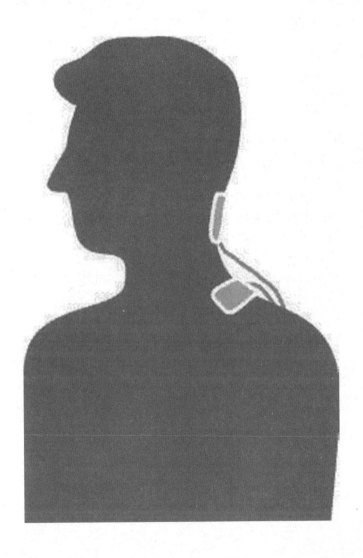

How magnets are used

Many types of magnet are available for therapeutic use, but the most convenient and useful are electromagnetic patches (Acumed) which can be applied to most parts of the body.

Magnets may be used in combination with other complementary or orthodox treatments to enhance their effectiveness.

How do I use electromagnetic patches?

The body maps in a later section of this book show the acupuncture points for some of the more common conditions that electromagnetic patches can help. You can either apply a patch directly over tender areas, or areas of pain, or select the nearest acupuncture point(s).

Take the oval Acumed patch, holding it by the white protective tab. Do not touch the adhesive surface.

Hold the patch leaf straight in front of you, with the magnet facing away from you. Tear the perforated, narrow strip on the edge of the leaf to reveal the self-adhesive plaster. This will enable you to peel off the entire plaster (with magnetic, copper and zinc).

Press the entire oval plaster over clean, dry skin at the selected acupoint or tender spot. Peel off the white tab and smooth down the patch. Press down firmly to ensure it has stuck to the

Acupoints on the head, face and neck

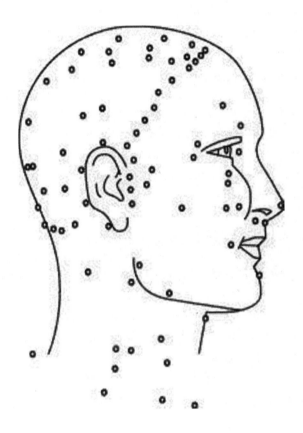

skin well. It is important the skin is dry, otherwise you will not obtain good adherence.

How many plasters can I wear at one time?

More than one plaster can be worn at the same time, depending on the spread and intensity of your pain.

Do I have to apply a patch over every acupoint illustrated?

No, these are only suggestions to show where traditional acupoints are sited. You can choose the point(s) you believe will help you best, or apply the patch directly over a tender area or the site of pain.

How long do I wear the plaster(s) for?

The optimum effect of magnet patch treatment is obtained between the third and fifth day. For reasons of hygiene, each patch should be used only once. If further treatment is required, use a new patch. Replace after 5 – 7 days, allowing the skin to breath.

Can I bathe while using Acumed?

You can safely bathe, shower or swim while using Acumed patches.

Acupoints on the arm

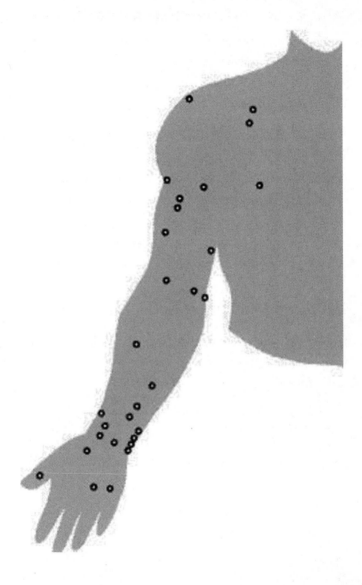

How do I remove Acumed patches?

All you need to do is gently pull the patch from the edges towards the centre. Any remaining adhesive can be removed with citrus-based skin cleansing lotion or tea tree oil.

How do I dispose of them?

Acumed patches are made from natural elements and function on natural forces. It has been observed that plants exposed to the south pole of a magnet grow more quickly. Earth worms are also driven away from the south pole. The south pole on the Acumed patches faces away from the skin. After using a patch, bury it in your garden in close proximity to your plants and in line with the earth's magnetic field.

When can I use another patch?

Allow the skin to breathe for a few days before applying a new plaster in the same spot. Make sure the skin is clean and dry when repeating the process.

Can I share a patch?

No. Never share or re-use the same patch for hygiene reasons.

Acupoints on lower leg

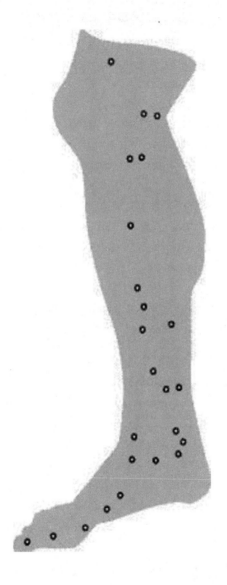

What conditions can benefit from magnetic therapy

Magnetic energy is one of the strongest natural forces on Earth, and many common conditions can benefit from magnetic therapy.

Some practitioners use single magnets, usually with the North pole in contact with the body, while others use an array of magnets aligned in rows or in concentric circles with the North (negative) and south (positive) poles alternating. This will result in many of the fields cancelling each other out, however, as their fields tend to flow towards the nearest opposite pole among adjacent magnets. Acumed patches, which consist of a rare earth magnet coated in zinc and surrounded by copper spheres, is the only system that provides both magnetic and electrical energy (See page 56) to provide a more powerful healing effect.

It is widely believed that the South or positive pole is stimulating and should not usually be used for healing when infection is present as it may stimulate growth of the invading bacteria or viruses as well. There is little evidence to back this up, however, and the World Health Organization have found that the strength of magnets commonly used for therapeutic purposes do not have any detrimental effects on health, which ever pole is used, as magnets provide a beneficial environment in which the body can heal itself to restore the correct balance between negative and positive energy fields within the body.

Acupoints on the leg

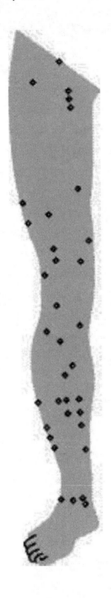

Magnetic patches can either be applied over sites of tenderness or pain, or applied to associated acupuncture points, as shown in the following illustrations. Select the points which most closely relate to the site of discomfort.

Unless otherwise stated, magnetic patches take three to five days to achieve full optimum effects. Wear the patch(es) for five to seven days, then discard. Rest the area for 2 days then, if necessary, reapply the patch(es) to continue treatment.

Pain

Pain is a sensation produced when small nerve endings, known as pain receptors, are stimulated in the body. It is an important symptom that alerts the body when something is wrong such as an injury, inflammation, infection or other disease. Because of the way nerve fibres join together as they travel through the body, the origin of pain is not always clear. Heart pain may be felt in the left shoulder or arm for example, gallbladder pain may be felt in the tip of the right shoulder, knee pain (eg arthritis) may seem to come from the hip while toothache may be felt in the ear.

Any pain that is persistent, severe, keeps recurring or which is accompanied by other symptoms should always be discussed with your doctor. Once the cause is diagnosed, and any appropriate treatment started, you can usually enhance the effect of therapy with the use of magnets assuming there are no contraidications (See page 84) such

Acupuncture points down the spine

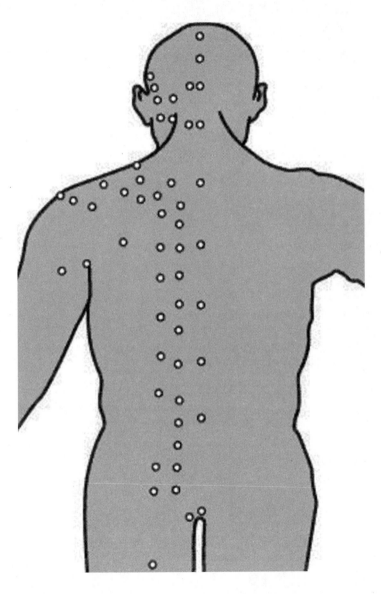

as the presence of infection. It is wise to let your doctor know you are using magnets.

Pain varies in a number of ways and may be described as:

- *Aching*
- *Burning*
- *Constant, intermittent or coming and going in waves*
- *Crushing*
- *Dragging*
- *Gnawing*
- *Throbbing*
- *Stabbing*
- *Stinging*
- *Superficial or deep*
- *Radiate to elsewhere in the body*

Do NOT use magnets to treat recurrent, undiagnosed pain.

Acupoints on back of leg

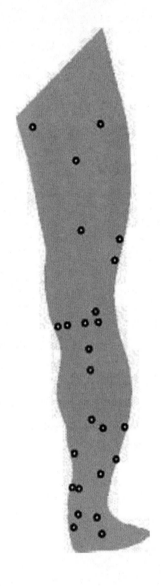

Magnetic therapy can help pain due to a number of causes, including

Backache	Menstrual pain
Burns (first degree)	Migraine
Carpal tunnel syndrome	Nervous tics
Constipation	Osteoarthritis
Cramp	Rheumatoid arthritis
Earache	R.S.I.
Erectile dysfunction	Sciatica
Fibrositis	Shoulder pain
Fracture pain	Sport injuries
Frozen shoulder	Tennis elbow
Gout	Tension Headache
Insomnia	Toothache
Jet lag	Travel sickness
Knee Pain	Whiplash
Keloid scars	

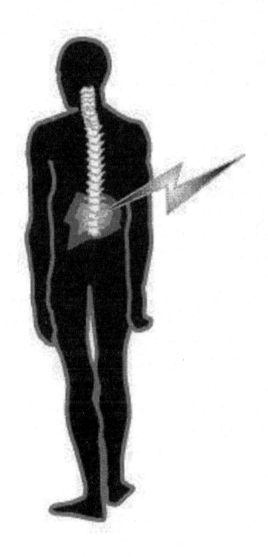

Backache

What it is

The spinal column is one of your body's main supports. It is made up of 33 small bones (vertebrae) that surround and protect the spinal cord. At the base of the spine, the 5 sacral vertebrae are fused to form the sacrum, and the 4 coccygeal vertebrae are fused into the coccyx (tailbone). In the upper part of the spine, the 7 cervical (neck), 12 thoracic and 5 lumbar vertebrae interlock in a series of sliding joints that give your backbone flexibility. These upper 24 vertebrae are separated from each other by pads of cartilage called intervertebral discs. These have a tough, flexible outer case with a soft, jelly-like centre and are designed to act as shock absorbers, cushioning the vertebrae from sudden jolts. Back pain most commonly affects the lower, lumbar region of the spine. Most cases are due to excessive strain on muscles, ligaments and small joints. As well as discomfort from the damaged tissues, the surrounding muscles may go into spasm so pain and tenderness spread over a larger area. More severe symptoms will occur if the soft, jelly-like centre of an intervertebral disc ruptures through the outer fibrous coating under pressure – a condition popularly known as a slipped disc. The prolapsed centre of the disc may press on the root of a spinal nerve to cause muscle weakness, pins and needles, spasm and pain in the back. If the sciatic nerve is irritated, pain will shoot down the leg (See Sciatica, page 174).

Spinal column

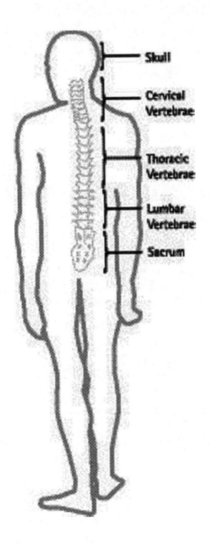

- Skull
- Cervical Vertebrae
- Thoracic Vertebrae
- Lumbar Vertebrae
- Sacrum

Back pain is most likely to affect people whose work involves heavy lifting or carrying, or who spend long periods of time sitting in one position or bending awkwardly. Almost any day to day activity can bring it on, however, including housework, gardening, and over-vigorous exercise. If you are overweight and unfit, with poor muscle tone, you are also at increased risk as apart from having to support a heavier load, your back will not receive the support it needs from your abdominal muscles.

Self help measures:
Try to lose any excess weight and improve your level of physical fitness.

Try to remain active, as early mobilisation is essential to stop your back seizing up.

Seek medical advice is back pain is persistent, severe, or if you develop numbness or weakness.

Applying magnetic patches
It is usually more effective to use two rather than one magnetic patch. For low back pain, try applying a magnet on either side of the spine (roughly four inches apart), in the small of the back, two fingerbreadths above the pelvic bone.

Magnetic patches can also be applied to acupuncture points over or near the site of pain, as shown in the following illustration. Select one, two or more of the points shown which most closely relate to the site of discomfort.

Acupuncture points for backache

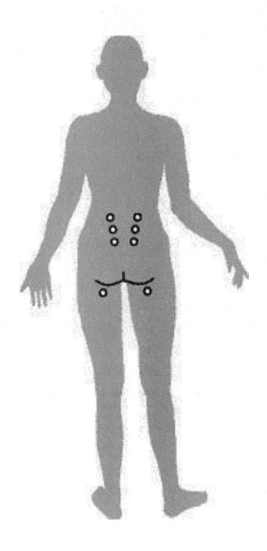

Burns

What it is

The skin is designed to protect the body from a variety of environmental insults, including excessive heat. If skin temperature rises above 49 degrees Centigrade, however, burning occurs. There are three levels of severity. In a first-degree burn, of which sunburn is the commonest cause, only the top layer of skin is damaged. This usually heals quickly with dead cells peeling after a few days. A second-degree burn causes damage to deeper layers of the skin and a blister typically forms. Enough live cells remain for skin to heal, however, and it does not usually scar unless the wound becomes infected. A third-degree burn is the most serious and involves damage to the full thickness of the skin. Extensive treatment, including skin grafts, may be needed and scarring is likely. If second or third degree burns cover more than 10% of the body area, fluid losses can result in clinical shock, in which the pulse speeds up, the blood pressure falls and the person collapses. Burns due to chemical or electrical damage can be deceptively deep and should always be checked by a doctor.

Self help measures:

Immerse the area in cold, running water, or soak a clean towel in cold-water and hold against the burn until pain eases. Dress the burn with a clean, non-stick, non-fluffy material such as sterile gauze. In an emergency, wrapping cling film round a large burn helps to prevent fluid loss.

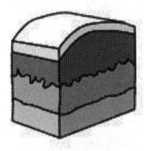

First Degree Burn

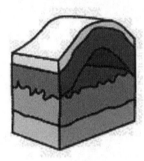

Second Degree Burn

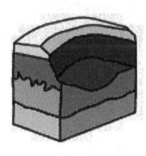

Third Degree Burn

Burns easily become infected – seek medical advice for all but the most superficial burns.

- Don't use adhesive plasters
- Don't apply butter, oil or grease
- Don't burst any blisters
- Don't try to remove any clothing stuck to the burn
- Don't use fluffy dressings (e.g. cotton wool)

Applying magnetic patches

Magnetic patches can also be applied over a first degree burn to hasten healing and reduce pain. Apply the patch to a piece of clean gauze, and place this immediately over the burn (do not stick adhesive directly onto burned skin). For larger areas, apply the patch to acupuncture points over or near the site of pain, as shown in the following illustrations. Select the points which most closely relate to the site of discomfort.

Do not use magnetic patches over areas that are raw, weeping or blistered.

Always seek medical advice for all but the most superficial burns.

Hand burn surrounded by possible magnets points

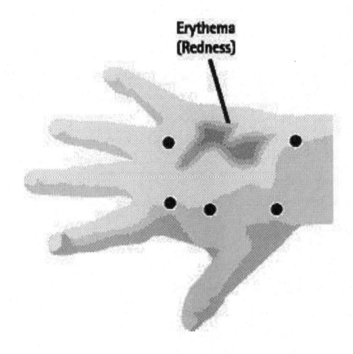

Erythema
(Redness)

Carpal tunnel syndrome

What it is

The carpal tunnel is a narrow space in the wrist that is formed where a strong ligament that connects the base of the thumb and little finger passes across the bones at the front of the wrist. The median nerve passes through this space, and carpal tunnel syndrome (CTS) occurs when the nerve becomes pinched to cause painful tingling in the hand, wrist and forearm. In severe cases, numbness, weakness and muscle wasting may occur. Symptoms classically affect the thumb, index and middle fingers and the inner side of the ring finger as these areas are supplied by the median nerve. Carpal tunnel syndrome is most commonly seen in middle aged women. It often affects both hands and is sometimes associated with obesity, pregnancy, underactive thyroid gland, fluid retention or repetitive finger movements (eg typing).

Self help measures:

Frequent work breaks are important.

An ergonomic assessment of work conditions is essential as altering posture, chair and table heights, computer-placement, and the correct use of a keyboard can improve symptoms.

Some people with CTS have a low vitamin B6 level (needed for optimum nerve functioning) and high dose supplements containing B6 are said to help at least 85% of people within 12 weeks. High dose vitamin B6 is best taken under

Carpal tunnel

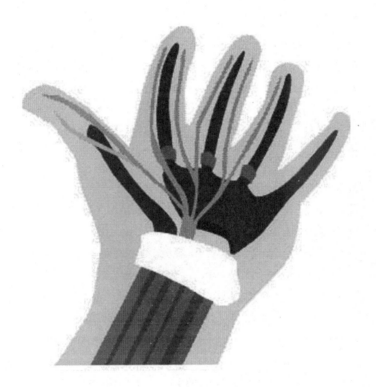

supervision of a nutritional therapist as excess may, in itself, lead to nerve conduction problems.

Applying magnetic patches
Apply two patches, one on either side of the wrist, above and below the most painful area.

Magnetic patches can also be applied to acupuncture points over or near the site of pain, as shown in the following illustrations. Select the points which most closely relate to the site of discomfort.

Constipation

What it is
Constipation is difficulty in passing motions, usually because they are too hard. Constipation may be diagnosed if you pass bowel motions less than twice a week, or if you have to strain to pass hard motions more than 25% of the time. Persistent constipation and straining at stool can also lead to a number of other problems including haemorrhoids, diverticular disease, anal fissures and even rectal prolapse which will in turn make constipation worse. Advanced age, side effects of some medications (eg codeine phosphate, iron), bowel obstruction (eg bowel tumour, scar tissue) and abnormal masses (eg large fibroid or ovarian cyst) can also be a cause.

If constipation is persistent, always seek medical advice.

Apply 2 patches, one on either side of the wrist,
above and below the most painful area

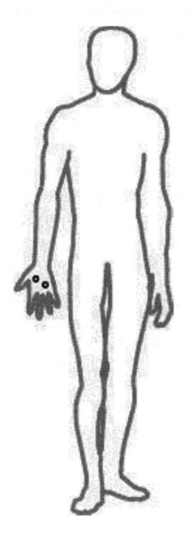

Self help measures:

Ensure a good intake of fibre-rich wholefoods such as brown bread, brown rice, wholegrain cereals, salads, fresh fruit and vegetables.

Drink plenty of fluids – especially mineral water – aiming for 2 to 3 litres of fluid intake per day.

Take regular brisk exercise

Do not put off visiting the bathroom when nature calls.

Psyllium seed/husks are a safe and effective remedy for constipation, increasing the frequency of bowel movements and making stools softer and easier to pass.

A probiotic supplement supplying friendly digestive bacteria will help to maintain healthy bowels.

Applying hot and cold compresses to your abdomen can help, especially if followed by an aromatherapy abdominal massage with diluted oil of Ginger (or if you prefer, use Lemon, Sandalwood, Mandarin, Orange, Grapefruit or Neroli). Massage the abdomen in a clockwise direction, starting on the lower left side.

Apply 5 magnetic patches in a V-shaped formation
just below the navel

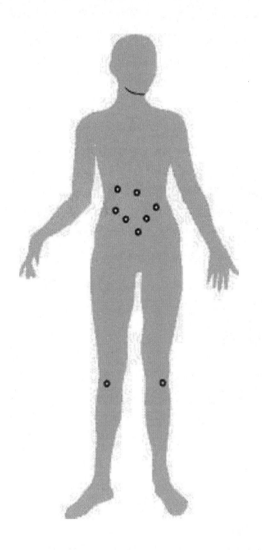

Prunes and prune juice are especially helpful as the fruit are a good fibre source (13% weight for weight) while the juice has a laxative action boosted by the presence of an hydroxyphenylisatin derivative similar to the laxative drug, bisacodyl, which stimulates secretion of fluid into the bowels and also stimulates intestinal contraction. They may cause flatulence initially, but if eaten regularly this effect improves as bowel bacteria adapt to producing more of the enzymes needed to digest the fibre they contain.

Applying magnetic patches

Apply five magnetic patches in a semi circle or V-shaped formation just below the navel (see previous page).

NB Do not use magnetic therapy during pregnancy.

Cramp

What it is

Cramp is a painful, excessive contraction of a muscle. This is usually felt in the leg, but any muscle can be affected. Cramps are linked to a build up of lactic acid and other waste products of muscle metabolism – usually during or after physical exercise. Cramp can also be triggered by repetitive movements (eg writer's cramp) and through sitting or lying in an awkward position. Poor circulation decreases the oxygen supply to muscles and interferes with the flushing away of lactic acids and other chemicals. This can happen at night in elderly people with hardening and furring up of their leg

Magnetic points for leg cramp

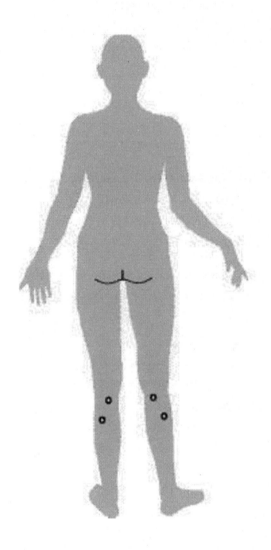

arteries. After eating a heavy meal, blood is diverted away from peripheral muscles to aid digestion – one reason why swimming immediately after eating is not advised. Excessive sweating, a fever, and hot weather can also cause cramps due to dehydration. If cramping lasts longer than an hour, seek medical advice.

Self help measures:
Ensure you drink plenty of fluids during the day, especially mineral water.

Increase your dietary intakes of calcium (eg low-fat milk, cheese, yoghurt etc, dark green leafy vegetables) and magnesium (nuts, seafood, dairy products, wholegrains, dark green, leafy vegetables).

Supplements that help to improve poor circulation include garlic tablets, omega-3 fish oil supplements or Ginkgo biloba extracts.

Coenzyme Q10 increases oxygen uptake in muscle cells and may also reduce the frequency of cramps.

Applying magnetic patches
Apply a magnetic patch over the centre of the cramping muscle. Patches can also be applied to acupuncture points over or near the site of pain, as shown in the following illustrations. Select the points which most closely relate to the site of discomfort.

Magnetic points for leg cramp

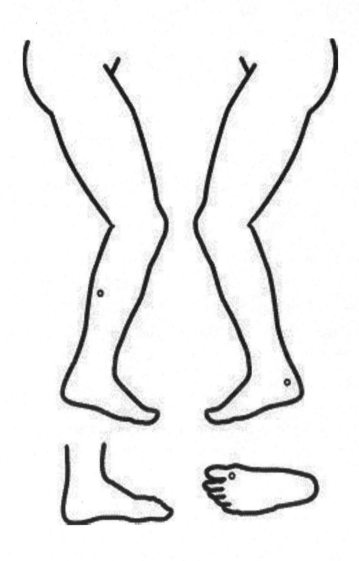

Earache

What it is

Earache is usually due to infection or inflammation of the outer or middle parts of the ear. This is usually due to a viral infection, but is occasionally bacterial. Symptoms can include earache, a feeling of fullness in the ear, reduced hearing, ringing or buzzing in the ear (tinnitus) and fever. Earache can also be due to a build up of wax, a boil in the ear canal, a build up of catarrh in the Eustachian tube, or infections elsewhere in the region such as tonsillitis, tooth abscess, or mastoiditis (infection of part of the bony skull behind the ear).

Self help measures:

If pain is not too severe, rest the ear against a warm hot-water bottle to ease pain.

If pain is severe, or discharge occurs, seek medical advice before using magnetic patches.

Applying magnetic patches

Apply a magnetic patch to the bony hairless area just behind the ear. Magnetic patches can also be applied to acupuncture points over or near the site of pain, as shown in the following illustration. Select the points which most closely relate to the site of discomfort.

Magnet points for earache

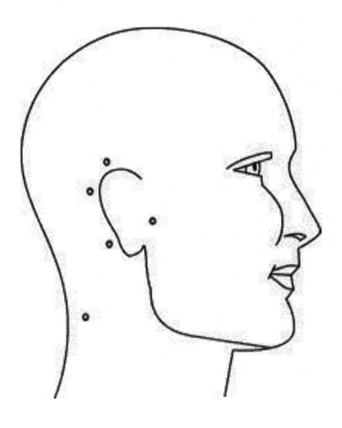

Erectile dysfunction

What it is

Impotence – known medically as erectile dysfunction – the persistent failure to develop erections that are firm enough for satisfactory sexual intercourse. It is a common and distressing problem, affecting an estimated 1 in 10 men at any one time. Although impotence can affect men of all ages – especially those who smoke – it becomes increasingly common in later life so that 40% of men aged 40 and almost 70% of those aged 70 years have some form of impotence.

Eighty per cent of all cases of impotence have an underlying physical cause. The most common physical causes of impotence include:

- *Diabetes - which can affect both the local circulation and nerve supply to the penis*
- *Hardening and furring up of the arteries (atherosclerosis)*
- *Smoking indirectly causes impotence by increasing the effects of other risk factors such as high blood pressure and atherosclerosis*
- *Long term abuse of alcohol or drugs such as marijuana, codeine, amphetamines and heroin can cause impotence.*
- *Prescription drugs – especially those used to treat high blood pressure, depression, heart disease, gastric ulcers and cancer*
- *Leaky veins in the penis*
- *Hormone imbalances*
- *Previous surgery that may have affected local blood circulation or nerve supply*
- *Spinal cord injury*
- *Some nervous system diseases such as multiple sclerosis, Parkinsonism, Alzheimer's disease and epilepsy*

Diagram of the Urolgic System

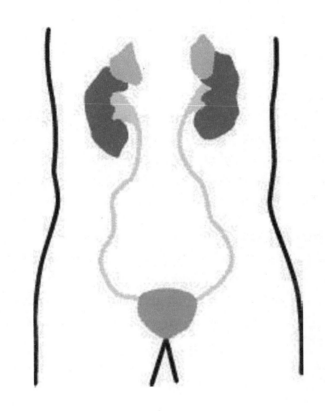

Psychological causes of impotence only account for one in five cases, and are often linked with depression. More commonly, psychological problems follow on as a result of the emotional stress of impotence. Over twenty per cent of sufferers blamed erectile dysfunction for the break up of their relationships.

If impotence is persistent, it is important to pluck up courage to seek help to find out the cause.

Self help measures:
A number of herbal supplements are effective in overcoming impotence for many men. These include Catuaba (Erythroxylon catuaba), Ginseng (Panax ginseng; P. quinquefolium), Muira Puama (Ptychopetalum olacoides) and Ginkgo biloba extracts.

Applying magnetic patches
Apply two magnetic patches in the midline between the navel and pubic bone. Another magnetic patch should also be applied at the front of each thigh, in the middle towards the inside over an acupoint as shown in the following illustration.

Fibrositis and fibromyalgia

What it is
Fibrositis is a non-medical term that means different things to different people. It literally means "inflammation

Magnet points for impotence

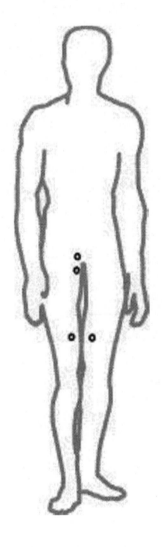

of fibrous tissue" and many doctors use it to describe minor aches and pains in muscles and joints for which they can find no obvious cause. Others use the term fibrositis to mean fibromyalgia (literally pain in muscle fibres) and the two terms are used interchangeably in some medical textbooks.

Fibromyalgia is a debilitating condition with widespread aches and pains plus sleep disturbance. Women are five times more likely to suffer than men. The pains tend to move from place to place, vary in severity and are often made worse by cold and stress. Sufferers develop localised areas of tenderness known as trigger points, especially around the lower spine, between the shoulder blades, at the base of the neck, over the sacro–iliac joints, elbows and knees. In some people, these tender spots develop fibrous nodules. Fibromyalgia seems to be due to reduced energy production in muscle cells and an inability of muscle fibres to relax. Sufferers do have a characteristic lack of delta wave (deep non-REM sleep) when brain waves are monitored during sleep, however. They therefore feel tired and exhausted much of the time as they wake unrefreshed. Interestingly, if normal volunteers are monitored during sleep and woken periodically so that they lack delta wave sleep, similar aches and pains will appear.

Self help measures:
St John's Wort will help where mild to moderate depression is present (check with a pharmacist if you are taking prescribed medication as interactions are possible eg with the oral contraceptive pill).

Brain waves during sleep

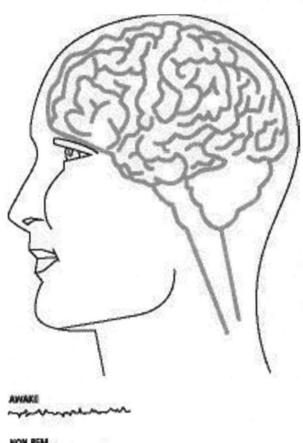

Supplements containing magnesium, B group vitamins, manganese and/or co-enzyme Q10 may help.

Relaxation techniques such as yoga, T'ai Chi and breathing exercises are beneficial.

Relaxing herbs such as valerian can improve sleep.

Gentle muscle massage and the application of heat can improve pain.

Applying magnetic patches

Magnetic patches can also be applied to acupuncture points over or near the site of pain, as shown in the following illustration. Select the points which most closely relate to the site of discomfort.

Fracture pain

What it is

Healing of a broken bone starts with the formation of a blood clot at the fracture site. Protein fibres known as fibrin form, which align themselves across the fracture site in a shape resembling a spindle which is sensitive to the magnetic field present. Calcium ions are then attracted to the fibrin and new bone formation builds up to form a callus which is slowly strengthened and remodelled over the following months. A bone normally has a positive magnetic polarity at the end closest to the centre of the body, and negative magnetic polarity at the end furthest from the centre of the body. This polarity is interrupted at the site of a fracture, however.

Magnet points

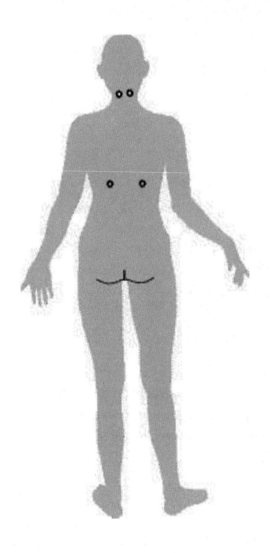

Self help measures:

Maintaining a good dietary intake of vitamins and minerals such as calcium, vitamin D and vitamin C which are important for bone health.

Applying magnetic patches

Restoring the correct magnetic field at the edges of the fracture hastens the healing process so that calcium ions can be laid down more readily. Bone fractures are sometimes found to heal in half the normal time when magnetic therapy is used.

Apply a magnet to either side of the bone fracture site. Magnetic patches can also be applied to acupuncture points over or near the site of pain, as shown in the following illustration. Select the points which most closely relate to the site of discomfort.

Frozen shoulder

What it is

Frozen shoulder is the common name for increasing pain, stiffness and immobility of the shoulder joint. It is due to inflammation and thickening in the lining of the capsule surrounding the joint (capsulitis). In most cases, no obvious cause is found, but it may come on after a fall, a task involving repetitive movements of the joint (eg painting the ceiling) or after unaccustomed exercise. Attacks have also been linked with other medical conditions such as chronic

Possible magnet points for leg fracture

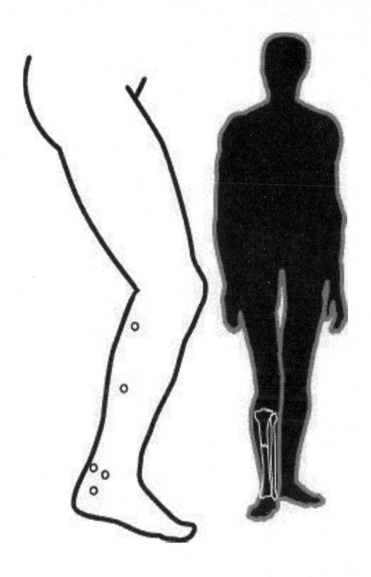

bronchitis, stroke or heart pain (angina), perhaps triggered by general immobility.

Self help measures:
During the initial, acutely painful stage of frozen shoulder, rest is usually advised.

Applying hot or cold packs can help.

After the pain starts to reduce, manipulation by a physiotherapist, osteopath or chiropractor will improve mobility, but it can take many months before the range of movement approaches normality again.

Applying magnetic patches
Apply one or more magnets over the most painful sites – relief often occurs within half an hour. Magnetic patches can also be applied to acupuncture points over or near the site of pain, as shown in the following illustration. Select the points which most closely relate to the site of discomfort.

Gout

What it is
Gout is an inflammatory arthritis due to high levels of uric acid which precipitate out into joints and tissues. This produces symptoms of a hot, red, swollen, exquisitely sensitive joint and usually affects the big toe, although any joints in the body can be involved.

Magnet points for frozen shoulder

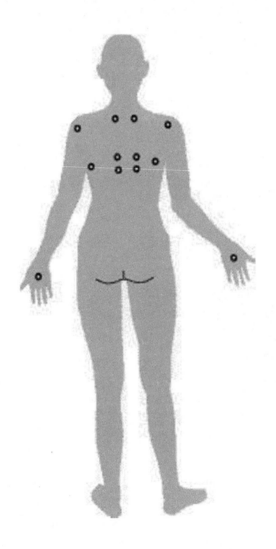

Self help measures:

Standard dietary advice is to reduce your intake of purine-rich foods such as offal, shellfish, oily fish, game, meats, yeast-extracts, asparagus, and spinach. Avoid alcohol as it both increases uric acid production and reduces its excretion – especially beer which is also rich in purines. As most uric acid is produced in the body during the breakdown of purines released when the genetic material (DNA) of worn out cells is recycled, however, dietary changes can only lower uric acid levels by up to 20%.

Applying magnetic patches

Apply a magnetic patch over sites of tenderness, or apply several patches to surround the area.

Magnetic patches can also be applied to acupuncture points over or near the site of pain. Select the points which most closely relate to the site of discomfort.

Insomnia

What it is

Insomnia is a difficulty getting off to sleep or in maintaining sleep. Most people need less sleep as they get older. While the average adult sleeps for between 7 and 8 hours per night, those over the age of 70 often only need 5 hours. Symptoms that can result from insomnia include tossing and turning without being able to get off to sleep, waking unusually early in the morning and not being able to get back to sleep, feeling

Magnet points for Insomnia

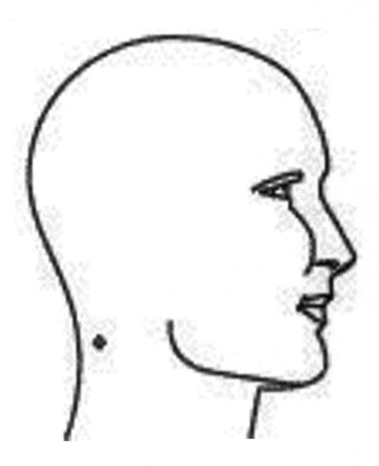

tired and listless during the day, yawning a lot, and feeling unusually irritable or snappy. Insomnia will also cause poor concentration and increase the risk of accidents.

Self help measures:
Take regular, brisk daily exercise but avoid strenuous exercise in the evening.

Avoid napping during the day

Avoid over-indulgence in substances that interfere with sleep such as caffeine (coffee, tea, chocolate, colas) nicotine, alcohol and rich or heavy food - especially close to bed-time.

Make sure your bedroom is comfortably warm, quiet and dark.

Applying magnetic patches
Apply a magnetic patch in the centre of the forehead, and another patch behind each ear (on the bony, hairless point two fingerbreadths behind the earlobe). The patches behind the ear can be left on continuously for up to 7 days, with the forehead patch just applied at night if you wish.

Jet Lag

What it is
Jet lag is a disturbance of the body's 24-hour sleep-wake biorhythms due to flying across several time zones, especially

Magnet points for Insomnia

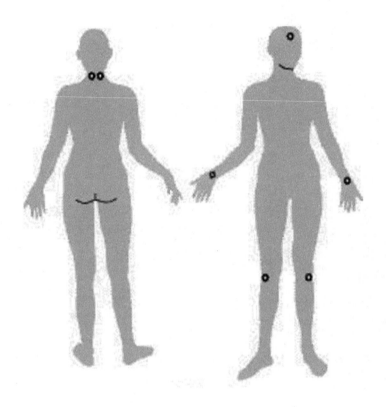

in an eastwards direction which shortens the traveller's day. Moving across the Earth's magnetic field from one pole to another may also play a role (See page 48). Jet lag is most likely to affect people over 30 who normally follow an established daily routine, causing symptoms of general disorientation, fatigue, poor memory, insomnia, headaches, irritability, poor concentration, decreased mental ability and reduced immunity.

Self help measures:
If flying east, try going to bed earlier than usual for several nights before traveling.

If flying west, stay up later than usual for several nights before leaving.

During the flight, drink plenty of fluids, avoid alcohol, only eat light meals and sleep as much as possible.

Take high dose antioxidants (eg vitamin C 1g – 3 g with bioflavonoids per day; vitamin E 400 i.u. daily) before, during and after travelling.

Also take high strength vitamin B complex (eg 50 – 100mg) twice a day during the flight and for the first 2 days after arrival.

Applying magnetic patches
Apply a magnetic patch to the centre of the forehead for half an hour once the plane has landed.

Magnet point for Jet Lag

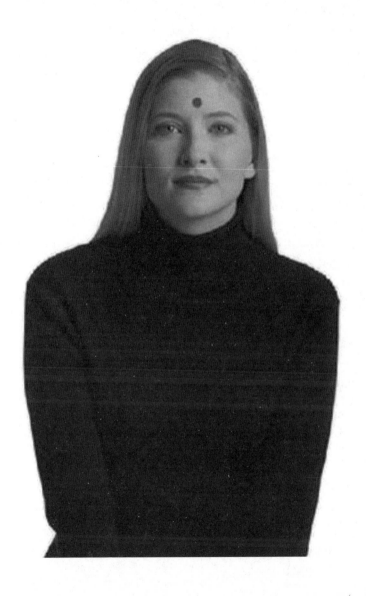

Keloid scars

What it is

Scars are formed as a part of the body's natural healing process in which damaged areas of skin are replaced by scar tissue - collagen - which shrinks and forms a pale scar. If the sides of the wound are well aligned and close together, the scar forms a thin white line but if the edges of the wound are separated or there has been extensive tissue loss, pink granulation tissue forms first which is then slowly replaced to form a tough, wide scar. Sometimes, an abnormally thickened area of scar tissue may form, due to an over-active healing response and the production of excessive amounts of collagen tissue. This is known as a keloid scar which is harder, more irregular and thicker than usual. The tendency to produce keloids can run in families and is most common over the trunk of the body.

Self help measures:

Rubbing in vitamin E oil/cream may help but some people develop a sensitivity reaction.

The appearance of scars – even old ones - can be helped by applying an adhesive gel sheet (from chemists) which helps to flatten, soften and fade scars that are red or raised.

Applying magnetic patches

Apply one or more magnetic patches over the keloid scar depending on its size – ideally as much as possible of the scar should be covered in magnets.

A post-operative keloid scar

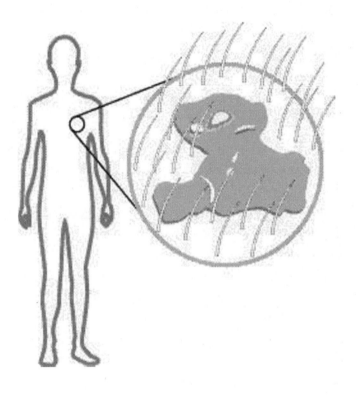

Knee pain

What it is

The knee is a modified hinge joint between the upper end of the tibia (shin bone), the lower end of the femur (thigh bone) and the patella (knee bone) at the front. Each bony surface is protected by slippery cartilage, and the joint lined with a synovial membrane which secretes fluid to oil and cushion knee movements. The ends of the tibia and femur are further protected by two crescent-shaped discs of cartilage, the medial and lateral menisci, that act like washers to reduce friction when the bones move together.

Strong fibrous bands of tissue hold the joint together, including the knee capsule, collateral ligaments at the side of the joint, plus two ligaments inside the joint itself (cruciate ligaments). These maintain stability and allow the joint to bend while stopping the ends of the bones from moving excessively back and forth or side to side. Strong muscles in the thigh attach to the bones via tendons near the knee joint and work together to move the joint. The hamstring muscles at the back of the thigh bend the knee, while the quadriceps muscles in the front of the thigh straighten it. Fluid filled sacs (bursas) above and below the knee help to prevent tendons and muscles from rubbing at pressure points.

Pain around the knee can be due to a number of conditions, including arthritis, sports injuries such as strained muscle,

Knee Pain

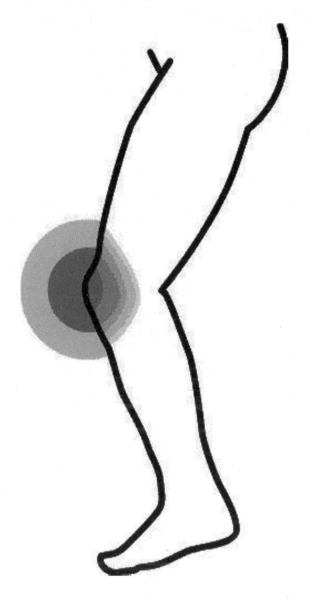

sprained ligaments or torn cartilage (meniscus) and bursitis (eg Housemaid's Knee).

The usual cause of a knee strain, sprain or torn cartilage is a sudden twisting movement when playing sport or during a fall. Soft tissue damage causes inflammation resulting in swelling, bruising, tenderness, stiffness and a reduction in mobility. The fluid-filled space surrounding the knee (bursa) usually also fills with inflammatory fluid (effusion) and cause dramatic ballooning of the joint. Immediate treatment is vital to minimise inflammation and swelling and to hasten healing. This will reduce the amount of time you are out of action.

Torn cartilage

The crescent-shaped medial and lateral menisci tear when a sustained, rotational strain is placed on a knee that is weight-bearing and flexed. This can cause a longitudinal split or a bucket-handle tear. Pain, swelling and instability occur initially, and later the knee may keep swelling, buckle, give way – especially when twisting – or "lock" so it can be flexed, but not fully extended when the torn piece of cartilage becomes trapped between the joint surfaces. Once a meniscus is torn, it will not heal as it does not have a blood supply. If the tear is removed, however, the meniscus may regenerate.

Knee Pain

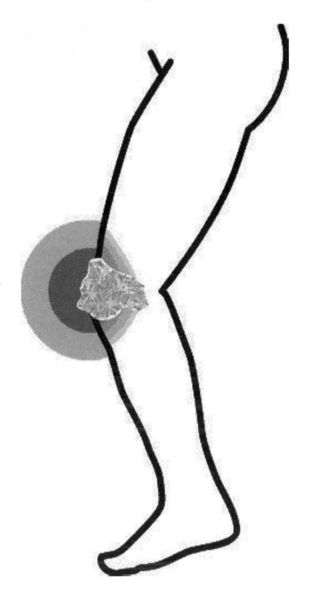

First Aid for Knee Injuries

Immediate treatment will minimise inflammation and swelling and hasten healing to reduce the amount of time you are out of action. To treat sprains and strains, just remember RICE:

> **R**est
>
> **I**ce
>
> **C**ompression
>
> **E**levation

Rest – for at least 24 hours to prevent further damage. Once pain and swelling start to subside, you may be able to start gentle exercise, but always follow medical advice. More severe injuries need to rest longer and may require immobilisation in a cast.

Ice: Apply an ice-pack (eg bag of frozen peas wrapped in a clean cloth) to the sprain or strain as quickly as possible to reduce bruising and swelling. Don't place ice directly on the skin as this can cause a cold burn. An ice-pack should only be applied for up to 10 minutes at time - remove for a few minutes before re-applying again if necessary.

Compression: An elasticated compression bandage will minimise swelling. This is best applied by someone with first aid training, as a bandage that is too tight will do more harm than good. Signs that a knee bandage is too tight include pins and needles, pain, blueness or numbness in the lower leg. Tubular compression supports are also available.

Knee Pain

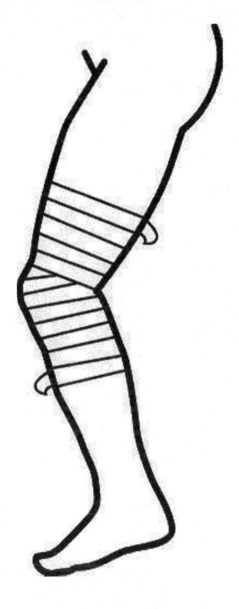

Elevate: Elevating the leg will reduce swelling eg prop your foot up on a chair with a cushion placed under the heel for support.

Anti-inflammatory painkillers – eg ibuprofen – by mouth or rubbed on in the form of a sports gel will help to reduce pain.

Seek medical advice if:

- Pain or swelling is severe.
- You think a muscle or ligament may be torn – eg if you can't bend a joint properly, or if a muscle seems to be oddly bunched or excessively painful.
- There is a flesh wound or bleeding – especially if your tetanus is not up-to-date.
- There is a possibility of a bone fracture (signs to look out for include bone tenderness with swelling, increased pain on movement and, in some cases, deformity).
- You are unsure how serious an injury is.

Further Self Help for knee pain

The knee joints have to work harder if you are overweight, so try to lose any extra pounds.

Exercises will help to reduce stiffness, improve mobility and strengthen the thigh muscles that stabilise the knee. A physiotherapist who specialises in sports' injuries can recommend individual approaches likely to get you back to work as soon as possible.

Supplements containing glucosamine sulphate are widely

Knee Pain

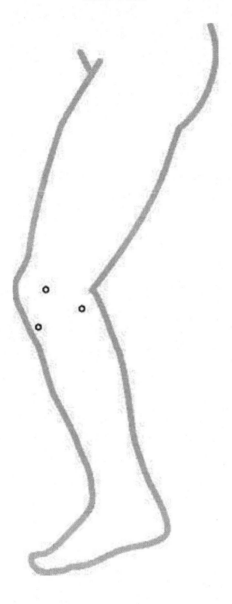

taken to supply building blocks needed for regeneration and repair of damaged joints, torn cartilage, sprained ligaments and strained tendons.

Extracts of the herb, Devil's Claw (Harpagophytum procumbens) are also used to help sports injuries by damping down inflammation and reducing pain.

Applying magnetic patches
Apply one or more electromagnetic patches over tender areas around the knee. Alternatively, apply a patch in the hollow behind each knee.

Menstrual pain

What it is
Menstrual pain (dysmenorrhoea) is due to excessive cramping of uterine muscles to produce pain during a period. This is most common in the first few years after menstruation starts, and again as the menopause approaches. Some women suffer more than others – possibly because they make more of the chemicals (prostaglandins) that trigger spasm of the womb wall. Another theory is that some women have an unusually narrow cervical outlet from the womb making cramping more likely before they have experienced pregnancy and childbirth. Painful periods can be triggered by conditions such as endometriosis, fibroids or polyps so if the problem is persistent or severe, do seek medical advice, especially if bleeding is heavy.

Self help measures:
Take gentle exercise (eg swimming) if you can manage it, as

Muscle points for menstrual pain

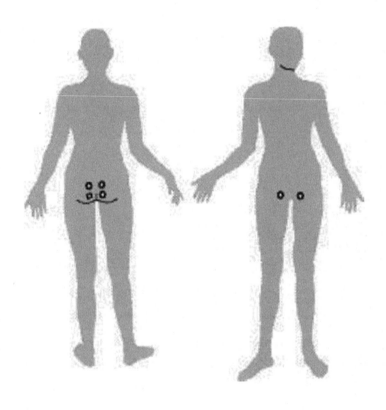

this encourages muscles to relax and triggers release of natural painkillers in your brain which can relieve period pains

Lie down somewhere quiet and cuddle a hot water bottle

Read a book, listen to music or watch T.V. to help take your mind off things.

Applying magnetic patches
Apply a magnetic patch at the mid point between the navel and the pubic bone.

Magnetic patches can also be applied to acupuncture points over or near the site of discomfort, as shown in the following illustrations. Select the points which most closely relate to the site of discomfort.

Migraine

What it is
Migraine is not just a headache, it is usually a full-blown attack. Symptoms are recurrent, with attacks coming on out of the blue and lasting from several hours to several days.

Migraine without aura - or common migraine - consists of a severe, throbbing, pulsating or hammering headache on one side, usually with abdominal symptoms. These include loss of appetite, nausea, vomiting, dislike of food, constipation or diarrhoea. 9 out of 10 sufferers experience this form of migraine.

Migraine with aura - or classic migraine - includes visual disturbances as well as any or all of the symptoms of

Magnet points for migraine

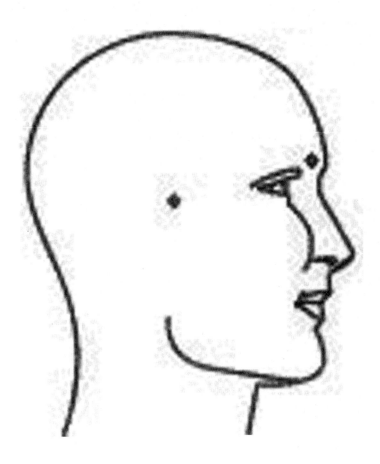

common migraine. Vision can be distorted with shimmering or flashing lights, strange zig-zag shapes or blind spots. 1 in 10 sufferers get this form of migraine.

Cluster headaches - attacks occur in clusters every 12 - 18 months. Severe pain is felt around one eye, often at night, for 1 - 3 weeks. The eye looks red and watery with engorged veins. The nose may become blocked up on the same side.

The exact cause of migraine is not fully understood. Attacks seem to be linked to chemical changes in the blood vessel walls and nerve cells within the skull. The most important chemical involved is called serotonin (5-hydroxytryptamine or 5HT for short). Migraine headache occurs when blood vessels widen so that tissues become congested. Serotonin is in short supply during this phase.

Self help measures:

Try to work out what factors trigger your attacks and, where possible, avoid them.

Common triggers include:

- stress or relief of stress (eg at the end of a long, trying week)
- physical fatigue or lack of sleep
- certain foods - eg cheese, alcohol - especially red wine, chocolate
- extreme emotions - eg anger, tension, excitement
- missed meals
- hormones eg menstruation, oral contraceptive pill.

Magnet points for migraine

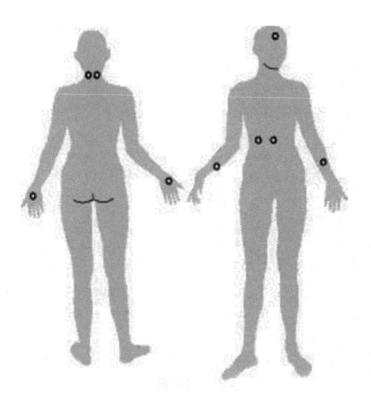

Applying magnetic patches

Migraine can often be relieved by applying a magnetic patch to the middle of the forehead. Once the migraine has gone, the patch may be removed.

Magnetic patches can also be applied to acupuncture points over or near the site of pain, as shown on the previous page. Select the points which most closely relate to the site of discomfort.

Nervous tics

What it is

A nervous tic is an involuntary, repeated contraction of one or more muscles. Nervous tics often develop in childhood and affect more boys than girls. Tics are often linked with stress, but the cause often remains unknown. Usually, the facial muscles are affected – classically around the eye – to produce repetitive blinking or mouth twitching, but nervous tics can also affect other parts of the body to cause uncontrolled movements of the limbs, shrugging of the shoulders, jerking of the neck, or vocalisations such as grunts.

Self help measures:

Counselling and stress reducing techniques may help.

Applying magnetic patches

Apply a magnetic patch over the affected muscle. Magnetic patches can also be applied to acupuncture points over or near the affected site, as shown in the following illustrations. Select the points which most closely relate to the area involved.

Magnet points for nervousness

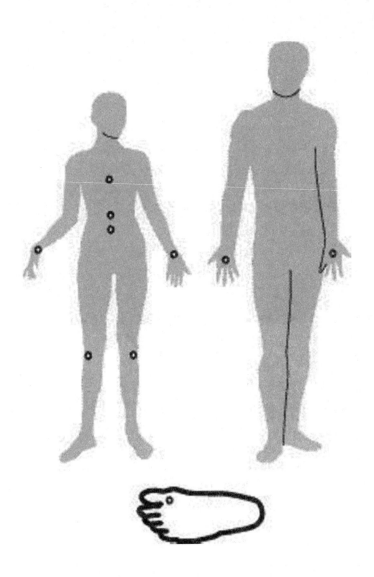

Osteoarthritis

What it is

The word arthritis means inflammation of a joint. There are many different forms of which the most common, osteoarthritis (OA), causes symptoms in at least half of people over the age of 60, and most others will have some X-ray evidence of the disease. OA usually affects the larger, weight bearing joints such as the hips, knees and spine but smaller joints eg the fingers and elbows can be involved too. The exact cause is not fully understood. It used to be thought of as a degenerative disease due to wear and tear on the smooth cartilage lining the joints, but is now believed to result from an active disease process. One theory is that imbalances occur in normal repair mechanisms so damaged cartilage is broken down and not properly replaced. This allows underlying areas of bone to rub together so affected joints becoming increasingly painful and stiff.

Self help measures:

Lose any excess weight.

Take regular, gentle exercise such as walking, cycling or swimming within the limits of discomfort, to maintain your strength and mobility.

Avoid walking over rough ground

Use a stick to reduce the weight load on joints

Apply hot or cold compresses – packs that you warm in the microwave or cool in the fridge are widely available from chemists.

Potent points for relieving arthritis

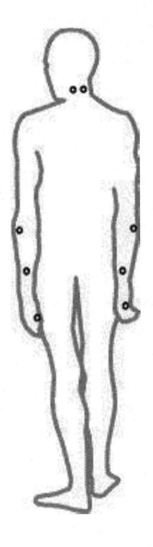

Sleep on a comfortable mattress that is not overly hard or too soft, both of which can make joint pain worse.

Supplements that can help include vitamin C, omega-3 fish oils, glucosamine sulphate, Devil's claw, New Zealand Green lipped mussel extracts, bromelain (pineapple extract)

Applying magnetic patches

Apply a magnetic patch over any painful joint. Magnetic patches can also be applied to acupuncture points over or near the site of pain, as shown in the illustrations on the previous page. Select the points which most closely relate to the site of discomfort.

Repetitive Strain Injury

What is it?

Repetitive strain injury (sometimes referred to as work related upper limb disorder) is an over-use condition that affects the muscles and tendons in the arms. Sufferers develop arm pains that are described as an ache or a cramping sensation, sometimes with numbness or tingling. Symptoms seem to be related to work, usually where fine repetitive movements of the fingers, hands or wrists occur. RSI is usually brought on by small, rapid, tense movements such as typing at a keyboard. When typing, tendons in the wrist slide to and fro inside their sheaths and if the wrist is held in an awkward position – cocked up, down or to one side – it can lead to inflammation of tissues around the sheaths (peritendinitis and tenovaginitis),

Repetitive Strain

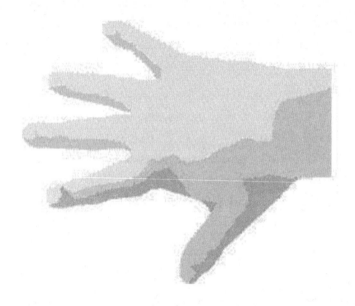

Seating Position

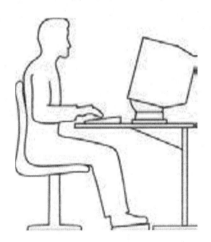

painful cramping in wrist, fingers or hands (writer's cramp) or inflammation of tissues surrounding a joint (eg tennis elbow). Carpal tunnel syndrome in which a nerve becomes trapped by tissue swelling in the wrist can also be made worse by certain work conditions.

People with work-related upper limb problems often develop pain that is difficult to pin down – there is no obvious sign of tissue injury or damage, which is why the term RSI – implying strain and injury is now considered a poor description. Some rheumatologists believe symptoms are due to a muscular condition, while others believe symptoms are associated with pressure on a nerve.

Unfortunately, recovery is often slow.

Self help
Rest is very important especially in the early stages. Physiotherapy can also help to build up strength of affected muscles, reduce pain using heat and ultrasound treatments and help to maintain limb mobility. Working splints may help, but are not always practical.

Prevention is terribly important – you can minimise the risk of upper limb pains by sitting with your body in the correct alignment and taking regular breaks.

- Take regular breaks from tasks requiring repetitive movements – try not to sit still for more than 20 minutes. Stretch arms back, upwards and forwards while sitting, and circle elbows to your sides.

Physiotherapy

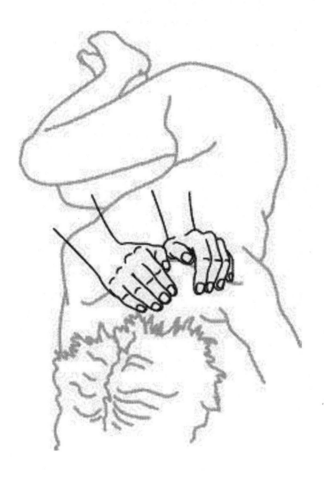

- Every hour walk around, swing your arms, touch your toes, jog on the spot etc to boost your circulation
- Make sure you sit correctly with back straight - don't sit cross-legged. You may find a seat wedge which tilts you forwards slightly is most comfortable
- When using a keyboard, your shoulders should be relaxed, your upper arm vertical, forearm horizontal and your wrist in a neutral, balanced position - not cocked upwards
- Your lower back should be supported at belt level
- Use ergonomically designed chair, VDU stand and wrist rest
- Keep feet flat on the floor or use a foot rest
- Use a document holder to minimise neck movements
- Ergonomically designed keyboards with specially shaped key pads and integral wrist rest are available
- Avoid excessive stress at work and try to minimise noise disturbance and interruptions when you are working
- The Japanese recommend that typists make no more than 40,000 key strokes per 8-hour day, yet bonus schemes in some UK companies depend on producing more than 10,000 keystrokes per hour.
- If you believe your work conditions are adversely affecting your health, contact the Health and Safety Executive who will arrange an inspection and keep your involvement anonymous so that your job is not at risk.

Acupoints on the hand

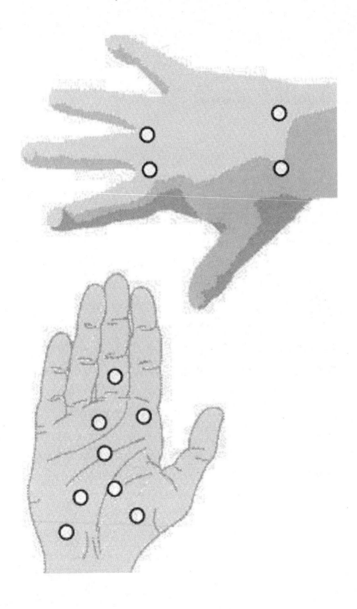

Applying magnetic patches

Apply one or more electromagnetic patches over tender areas on the arm or wrists. Easy to apply magnetic wrist bands are also available.

Rheumatoid arthritis

What it is

Rheumatoid arthritis (RA) is an inflammatory disease in which the synovial membranes lining some joints become thickened, inflamed and produce excess synovial fluid leading to redness, stiffness, swelling and pain. Inflammation gradually spreads to involve the underlying bone which becomes worn and distorted. Usually, RA affects the smaller joints in your hands and feet but can also occur in the neck, wrists, knees and ankles. People suffering from RA often feel unwell and may notice weight loss, fever and inflammation in other parts of their body such as the eyes. RA affects around 1% of the population, with three times as many women affected as men. A quarter of patients develop symptoms before the age of 30, but most new cases occur in the 40 - 50 age group. RA is now believed to result from the build-up of a type of immune cell (T-lymphocyte) that attacks the joints leading to inflammation and damage.

Self help measures:

Avoid cold draughts and keep as warm as possible in winter.

Magnet points for ankle pain

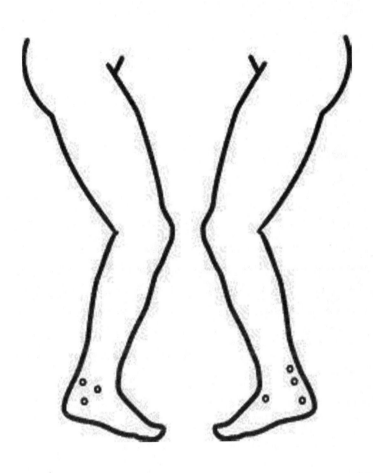

If hands are stiff in the morning, exercise them in hot, soapy water first thing in the morning and throughout the day. Frequent hot baths/showers are also soothing.

Some people find hot or cold compresses helpful.

Applying magnetic patches
Magnetic patches can also be applied to acupuncture points over or near the site of pain, as shown in the following illustration. Select the points which most closely relate to the site of discomfort.

Sciatica

What it is
Sciatica is a pain felt in the buttock and down the back of one leg, which occurs when the sciatic nerve is compressed or damaged. It is a common problem with most people experiencing it at least once during their life. The left and right sciatic nerves are the largest nerves in the body and run from the base of the spine, one down the back of each leg where they divide above the knee into branches that supply the lower leg and foot. Usually, sciatica only affects one leg, but in more serious lower back injuries, it may be bilateral.

Sciatica causes mild to severe pain felt in the buttock and/or down a leg. Pain may be continuous, or recurrent and is made worse by moving or coughing. Pain may be accompanied by tingling, skin numbness or muscle weakness and, if compression or injury to the sciatic nerve(s) is severe, you may be unable to life your foot on the affected side, or even to stand upright or walk.

Sciatica pain

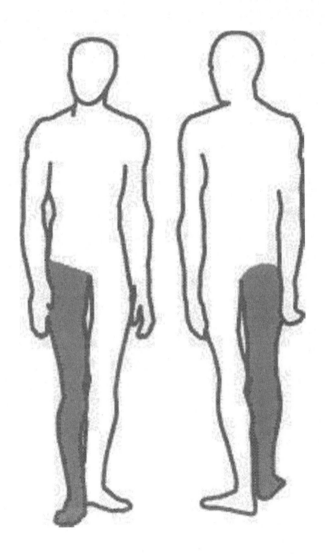

The usual cause of sciatica in those aged 20 to 40 years is a prolapsed (slipped) intervertebral disc which presses on the root of the sciatic nerve where it joins the spinal cord. Often, the cause of sciatica remain unknown, but latest research suggests some cases may be catching - scientists believe they have found evidence that shows that sciatica can develop from a bacterial infection. More than half of those studied were infected with a micro-organism that also causes acne.

Causes

Most cases of sciatica are due to a slipped disc. Other possible causes include:

- *a slipped vertebral bone (spondylolisthesis)*
- *osteoarthritis (in which bone spurs may develop on vertebrae)*
- *a growth such as a spinal tumour*
- *an abscess*
- *blood clot*
- *an injury (eg fractured pelvis)*
- *muscle spasm which increases pressure around the nerve such as when sitting in an awkward position for a prolonged period of time (eg travelling in cramped conditions)*
- *postural changes occurring during pregnancy*
- *a neurological disorder.*

Self help measures:

If you suspect you have sciatica, you should always seek medical advice for a full neurological examination of the legs and, if necessary, medical investigations and treatment.

Magnet points for sciatica

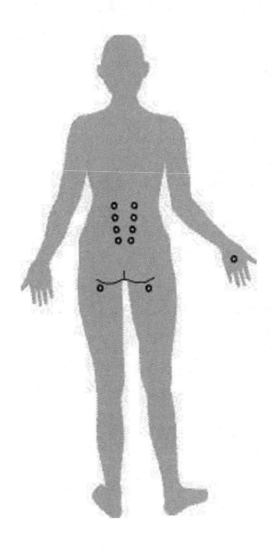

Applying magnetic patches

Magnetic patches can be used to hasten healing and reduce discomfort and can complement any treatment your doctor feels is necessary. Apply magnetic patches on either side of the lower spine – either over an area of pain or tenderness in the back, or in the small of the back. These can be aligned to form two rows of between one and four patches on each side, depending on the severity of the pain. At the back of the leg, apply another patch to the top of the affected thigh in the midline, just below the buttock, and another patch in the centre of the back of the knee.

Magnetic patches can also be applied to acupuncture points over or near the site of pain, as shown on the previous page. Select the points which most closely relate to the site of discomfort.

Shoulder pain

What it is

Non-specific shoulder pain may be due to muscle tension or spasm in the shoulder region, or to inflammation of the shoulder joint.

Self help measures:

Avoid heavy lifting

Check your shoulders are held straight, rather than rounded.

When sitting, keep back straight and shoulders back.

Magnet points for shoulder pain

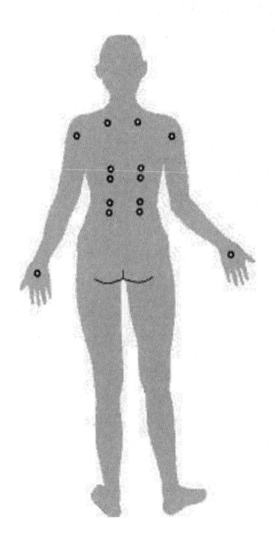

Applying magnetic patches

Gently feel over the shoulder, upper back and lower neck areas, and apply magnetic patches over any pressure sensitive/tender spots.

Magnetic patches can also be applied to acupuncture points over or near the site of pain, as shown in the following illustration. Select the points which most closely relate to the site of discomfort.

Sport injuries

What it is

Sports injuries are common among those who exercise regularly - especially if they are unfit and haven't warmed up properly. Even seasoned athlete's can run into problems however. Of all the sports played, rugby is the most dangerous when it comes to risk of sports injury. The Sports Council have previously found there was an average of only 20 consecutive rugby games or training sessions free of significant injury per player, compared with 76 injury-free sessions for soccer, 313 for badminton and 1,430 for keep-fit activities such as weight training, running and aerobics. Half the injuries were muscle strains and ligament sprains. Injuries seem to be fairly evenly distributed between the arms, ankles, legs, knees and back.

A strain is caused when a muscle is overused or suddenly overstretched so the muscle fibres pull apart or tear. This

Ankle sprain

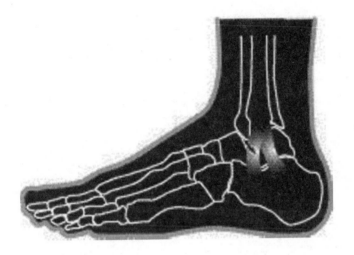

is more likely if you haven't warmed up before exercise of if your muscles are tense or fatigued. In severe cases, the muscle may rupture altogether.

A sprain is caused when a ligament – the tough, fibrous tissue that holds the bones of a joint together – is overstretched or torn. A sprain usually results in rapid swelling of the involved joint, most commonly the ankle or knee. In severe cases, the ligament may rupture altogether.

Strains and sprains usually result from a sudden twisting movement or fall. Tissue damage causes inflammation and produces symptoms of pain, tenderness and swelling. Bleeding into the area often results in bruising. Even mild strains and sprains can result in stiffness and reduced mobility unless they are treated promptly to minimise inflammation and swelling and hasten healing.

Self help measures:
To treat minor strains and sprains, just remember RICE:

> **R**est
>
> **I**ce
>
> **C**ompression
>
> **E**levation

Rest – minor injuries can usually be exercised within the limits of pain. You may need to rest for 24 hours to prevent further damage. Once the pain has subsided, you can usually start to exercise gently.

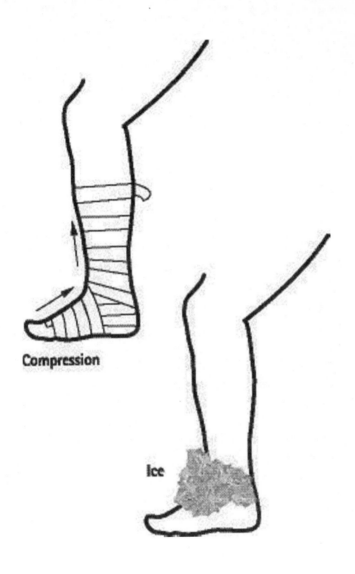

Compression

Ice

Ice: Apply an ice-pack (eg bag of frozen peas wrapped in a clean cloth) to the sprain or strain as quickly as possible to reduce bruising and swelling. Don't place ice directly on the skin as this can cause a cold burn. An ice-pack should only be applied for up to 10 minutes at time - remove for a few minutes before re-applying again if necessary.

Compression - apply a tubular compression support to minimise swelling when joints such as the ankle or knee are injured. These are available from pharmacies.

Elevate: If possible and practical, elevate the injured part to help reduce swelling eg prop up a twisted ankle on a chair (with a cushion placed under the heel rather than your calf) or wear a sling to elevate an injured wrist to shoulder level.

Applying magnetic patches
Gently feel over the sprained or strained area, and apply magnetic patches over any pressure sensitive/tender or swollen spots.

Magnetic patches can also be applied to acupuncture points over or near the site of pain, as shown in the following illustrations. Select the points which most closely relate to the site of discomfort.

Tennis elbow

What it is
Tennis elbow (epicondylitis) is a pain near the elbow caused

Magnet points for ankle sprain

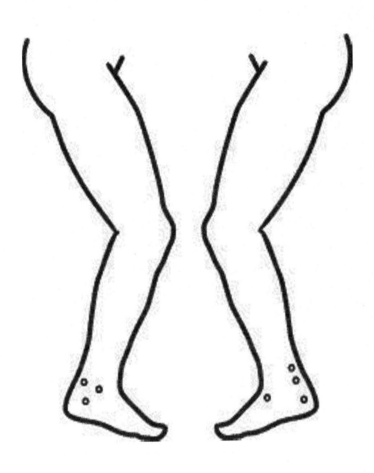

by inflammation where a tendon from the forearm muscles attaches to the bone. The inflammation results from overuse of the muscle and is especially common from racquet games when the grip is faulty. Gardening and heavy lifting can also bring it on. Symptoms include pain and tenderness on the outside of the elbow and the back of the forearm.

Self help measures:
Rest the arm for a couple of weeks

Apply an ice pack regularly (wrapped in cloth and only applied for up to 10 minutes at a time).

Applying magnetic patches
Apply one or more magnets over the most painful sites – relief often occurs within half an hour. Magnetic patches can also be used to surround the painful area, or applied to acupuncture points over or near the site of pain, as shown in the following illustration. Select the points which most closely relate to the site of discomfort.

Tension headache

What it is
A tension headache usually feels like a severe, continuous pressure on both sides of the head, which may centre over the top of the skull, the back of the head or above both eyes. Some tension headaches feel like a tight, constricting band, while others are more like a non-specific ache. Tension headache is often brought on by feelings of excess pressure,

Magnet points for tennis elbow

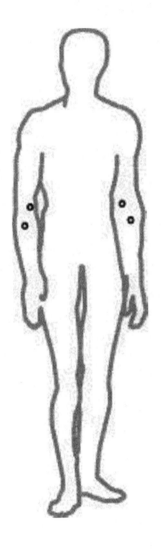

relief of stress (eg at the end of a long, trying week), physical fatigue, lack of sleep, missed meals and extreme emotions such as anger and excitement.

Always seek medical advice if headaches are persistent, severe or recurrent.

Self help measures:
To avoid muscle tension, try not to stoop when standing or sitting, concentrate on keeping your back straight, your shoulders square and your abdomen lightly pulled in.

Don't hunch your shoulders - hold shoulders straight yet relaxed – circle your shoulders from time to time, and don't fold your arms tightly – let them hang loosely from your shoulders, and shake your arms and hands regularly.

Avoid clenching your fists - hold hands loosely with your palms open and your fingers curled lightly and naturally, and don't clench or grind your teeth - keep your mouth slightly open and try to relax your upper and lower jaws.

Massage is often effective, as gentle manipulation of muscles in the neck, shoulders and back will relax taught muscles. This can be combined with relaxing aromatherapy essential such as camomile, geranium, lavender or peppermint.

Applying magnetic patches
Tension headache can often be relieved by applying a magnetic patch to the middle of the forehead. Once the headache has gone, the patch may be removed.

Magnet points for tension headache

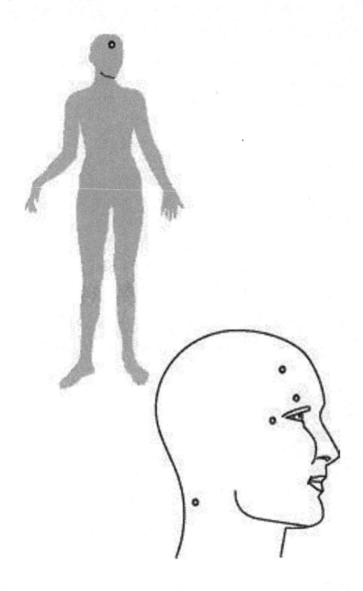

Alternatively, apply two patches at the base of the skull, where it joins the neck at the back. These are more discreet can be left in place for longer if you wish.

Magnetic patches can also be applied to acupuncture points over or near the site of pain, as shown in the following illustrations. Select the points which most closely relate to the site of discomfort.

Toothache

What it is
Toothache is a persistent, unpleasant, gnawing ache that is extremely distracting. Urgent dental treatment is needed, but while awaiting for your appointment, try applying a magnetic patch to the skin over the area of pain.

Self help measures:
Avoid eating or drinking food/fluids that are too hot or too cold.

Apply a little oil of Cloves to the affected tooth and massage into the surrounding gum to help numb the pain.

Applying magnetic patches
Magnetic patches can also be applied to acupuncture points over or near the site of pain, as shown in the following illustrations. Select the points which most closely relate to the site of discomfort.

Magnet points for toothache

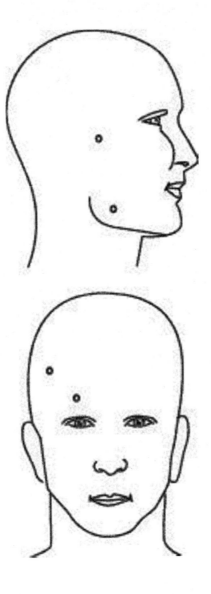

Travel sickness

What it is

Travel sickness occurs when your brain receives conflicting messages from your eyes and ears about the degree of movement experienced. This usually happens when travelling in a closed space (eg car, plane, below deck) when you tend to focus on nearby objects. Your eyes then tell the brain you are stationary, while your balance organs say you are not. Motion sickness is made worse by fear, anxiety, exhaust fumes, a stuffy atmosphere, a-full stomach and the sight or smell of food.

One in three people are highly susceptible to travel sickness, one in three only suffer during fairly rough conditions while the remainder only react in prolonged, violently rough situations. Mild symptoms include uneasiness, headache, dizziness and drowsiness. More severe symptoms include excessive sweating and salivation, vertigo, an irresistible desire to stop moving, nausea and profuse vomiting.

Self help measures:

Sit or stand near a source of fresh air when travelling

Sit between the wheels in a coach, or over the wings in an aeroplane

Eat little and often while travelling and avoid drinking alcohol

Focus on a distant point such as the horizon

Magnet points for travel sickness

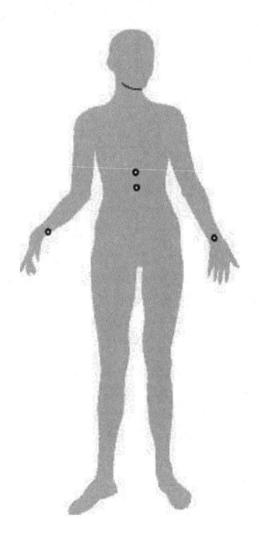

Avoid reading a book or looking at a map in the car

Take regular breaks to stretch your legs, if possible.

Applying magnetic patches

Apply a magnetic patch over the acupuncture point on each wrist. You can also apply a patch just under the rib cage in the midline at the front.

Whiplash

What it is

Whiplash is an injury to the neck commonly caused when sitting in a car that is either shunted in the rear, or which hits an object at the front. Although the body is strapped in, the head is not restrained and sudden acceleration or deceleration will jerk the head backwards and then forwards (or vice versa) to overstretch tissues in the neck. This leads to sprained or even torn ligaments, strained muscles and sometimes a partial dislocation of one or more of the small joints between cervical vertebrae.

Typically pain and stiffness increase over 24 hours following the original injury. Whiplash can also injure nerve fibres, leading to numbness, burning and tingling in the fingers and, in severe cases, may cause weakness or even paralysis of arm muscles. Other symptoms that may appear include headache and tinnitus (ringing in the ears).

Whiplash usually recovers fully, but it may be several weeks before full pain-free neck movements to return.

Whiplash

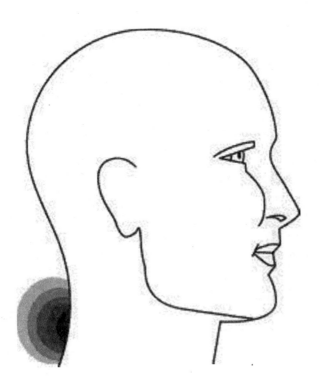

Self help

Applying a cold/ice pack during the first 48 hours, then switching to a moist heat pack (available from pharmacies).

Wearing a soft orthopaedic collar to support the weight of the head; this rests the neck muscles and ligaments allowing them to heal. Collars are usually only worn for a few days however so that muscles do not become overly weakened.

It will help to sleep on your back and to use a flat pillow so your head is not raised above your neck. Some people prefer lying curled on their side, but avoid lying on your stomach.

Supplements containing glucosamine sulphate help to boost repair of damaged ligaments, while antioxidants help to reduce inflammation.

Applying magnetic patches

Apply one or more electromagnetic patches over tender areas around the neck. Alternatively, apply two patches at the front of the neck and two at the back of the neck, at the level of maximum discomfort.

Easy to apply magnetic neck bands are also available.

Whiplash

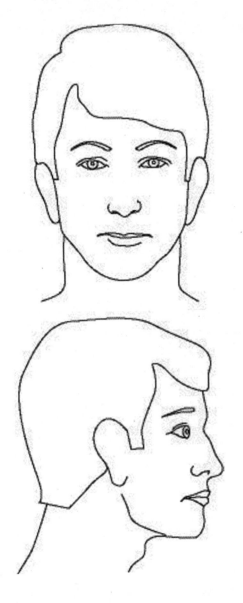

User Testimonials

In their own words from people who have used magnetic therapy patches.

"I have just tried the Magnetic patches pain patches and I am very impressed. Since I broke my right shoulder a couple of years ago the surgeon told me I would be prone to rheumatism or other aches eventually. The last couple of weeks I've experienced pain in my foot and knee. I've had tablets and creams from the doctor which didn't work. I saw these patches in the chemists, and tried them this week and I've felt more comfortable and less pain. Thank goodness. So I am pleased to tell you that they do work and I will use them again."

I. H.

"I saw the Magnetic patches advertised on the internet while looking for some pain relief for my husband. He has suffered from Sciatica and low back pain for nearly 20 years. He has had three operations, the last one two years ago was a spinal fusion, but he is no better. A year ago he retired through ill health at 50 years old. He has had an acupuncture kit for about 12 years and finds he does get some relief from that so when I told him about the patches he decided to try them. That was a week ago, and by the third day of using 3 patches on various acupuncture points the difference was amazing! He was moving easier and even went for a bike ride, which is virtually unheard of these days. Only a few days earlier he had been in bed because of the pain. So all I can say is THANK YOU for giving me my husband back again!"

Mrs M. S. R.

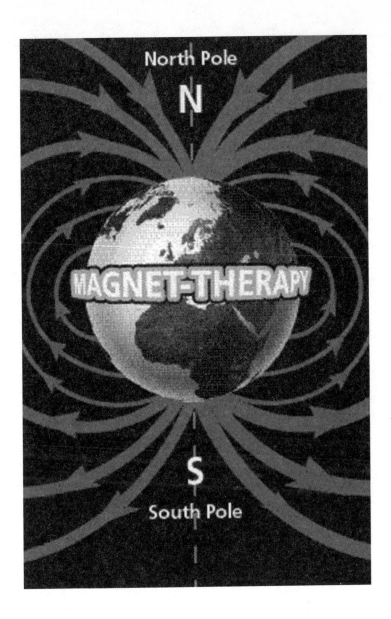

"I really must write to say how thrilled I am after only two weeks of using the pain patches for my lower back pain. The pain relief really has to be experienced to be appreciated. I know my arthritis will not be cured by the patches, but at least I can enjoy moving about so much more easily. THANK YOU."

Miss C. T.

"I ordered Magnetic patches for my husband – arthritic hole in the knee – started taking last year and he is almost pain free – he is a hotelier and on his "pins" all day, especially Christmas and New Year – first festive season without pain for 7 years! I have now recommended to 3 people, one of whom I spoke to today, who, at 33 had two sports damaged knees and in constant pain – he went for a run last week, for the first time in over a year! They work incredibly well."

Mrs D.

"I am writing to tell you that I have found your patches very effective in treating pregnancy nausea. About an hour after I had put them on, the nausea diminished a lot more than if I did not have them on at all.

I also used the patches when I wasn't pregnant for a back pain problem that I had and they helped them too.

It is great to find something that isn't medicinal and that is safe and natural and easy to apply yourself. THANK YOU."

S. C.

"I have just found and started to use the Magnetic Patches Pain Patches and would like to let you know how much they have helped me. I have had a bad hip and lived on medication, especially at night when sleep was a real nightmare and then the mornings leaving me very drowsy and slow to motivate – I spoke to the Pharmacist at Boots who recommended I see my doctor, as hip replacement has been my next option after pain killers. As I was walking out of the Prescription area I saw the box of patches and from then on my life changed from day one. I then introduced them to my daughter who has an Arthritic knee and she had the same wonderful relief. Thank you for this product."

Mrs A.

"I used Magnetic Patches Pain Patches on a recent long haul to New Zealand and followed your advised instructions with unbelievable results – a pain free flight over and back ... I have recently suffered with my right knee. I felt desperate for something to stop the pain and give me confidence to cope with the journey. I wouldn't hestitate to use these patches again and wouldn't ever think of ever flying without them. Many Thanks from a very satisfied customer."

Mrs T.

"I just wanted to say I had a dislocated knee from a football incident, which needs an operation or 2 due to damage to my ligaments and cartilage so I thought I would give your patches a go. Well they are brilliant, I went from absolute agony about 80% of the time, to just mild pain now."

Mr D.

"I just had to write and tell you how marvellous I have found your

Magnetic Patches patches. I have suffered with Sciatica, being unable to bend or rise from a chair without pain and assistance. Half way through my first Magnetic Patches pack, I can now sit down and get up without even using the arms of the chair – it is like being in someone else's pain free body. With a patch in each of two of the points you suggest for sciatica, I can bend and touch my toes, turn over in bed without the pain waking me. I will never be able to thank you enough."

Mrs S. D.

"I have been suffering intermediate back ache since an accident 14 years ago. However I managed to 'do something to it' whilst trying to remove a tree stump a few weeks ago. So whilst in Boots on Friday I decided to try 'something different', namely Magnetic patches. Now I can't say if the pain would have vanished naturally, if it was psychosomatic, or the thought of having parted with £12 for a box; or indeed that they really did something. But I spent the first weekend in nearly six weeks with little pain.

I'm normally sceptical (I trained as a scientist) but am amazed!"

Mr C.

"I've just bought a first box of *Magnetic Patches Pain Patches*. I have Osteoarthritis of the knee and have had a complete right side hip replacement in December through this. I would like to say how beneficial and comfortable they are! I wish I had known about them earlier. I wouldn't hesitate to recommend these to friends. I would be willing to partipate in any evaluations of this, or any other products. I-am 53."

Mrs H.

"I have found these very successful and after months of tennis elbow and pain, within a few days, I have had great relief and much less discomfort.

I am also prepared to participate in any evaluations of this or any other products."

S. J. H.

"Just a line to let you know how pleased I am with the loss of pain in my back.

I fell about 4 months ago and squashed a vertebrae, and have a small fracture in the spline. I put two of your patches on the area, and I am quite pleased with the result.

A friend of mine also had a great pain in her shoulder, and I gave her a patch to help. I have just talked to her, and she too is quite pleased with the result!"

Mr A. T.

"I would like to confirm, on using Magnetic Patches Pain Patches, for the first time, how I found them of much benefit on a recent long haul flight.

I suffer from Osteoarthritis of the knees, so felt and gained much relief of pain which is always much worse when flying – usually.

I would like to hear more information and wouldn't hesitate to use them again, or when the pain is worse – especially in wet winter days."

Mrs D. R.

"Magnetic Patches Patches are the best treatment I have ever used for the treatment of period pain. 100% effective and no side-effects ... perfect!!!"

Miss A. S.

"I am just writing to say how good the above product is. I have a arthritic condition of the knee. I can now walk and sleep without pain. I would be happy to participate in this on other products."

Miss G. A. P.

"I have had a bad pain in my back for a very long time. My doctor tells me it's a muscle and I need to rest as much as possible. I am greatfull for the relief I get from the patches. I thought you would like to know this."

Mrs A. J.

"I went on holiday a few weeks ago, and took along two packets of Magnetic Patches I picked up in Boots.

I have been having very painful bouts of Osteoarthritis in my joints and spline, having treatment from an Osteopath. I tried the patches and was amazed at the almost instantaneous relief. Imagine my surprise when I returned to find amongst my mail the special offer for Magnetic patches.

I will never be without them now. And hope I am finished with pain killers!"

Mrs L. F.

"Thank you for your letter of 23/04/01 also the Magnetic Patches Patches it was very kind of you to send them to me, I'm sure you will be pleased to hear that my knee is improving daily. I am enclosing an article from our Evening Standard newspaper and feel sure it will be of interest to you."

Mrs V. W.

Useful addresses

ACUMED
MAGNETIC THERAPY PATCHES
113 Pope Street, Birmingham B1 3AG
Tel: 44 (0)121 236 2073   Fax: 44 (0)121 233 4516
www.acumed.co.uk   email: info@acumed.co.uk

ARTHRITIS CARE
18 Stephenson Way, London NW1 2HD
Tel: 080 8800 4050

ASSOCIATION OF NATURAL MEDICINE
19 Collingwood Road, Witham, Essex CM8 2DY
Tel: 01376 502762

BACKCARE
16 Elmtree Road, Teddington, Middlesex TW11 8ST
Tel: 0208 9775474

BRITISH COMPLEMENTARY MEDICINE ASSOCIATION
PO Box 5122, Bournemouth BH8 0WG
Tel: 0845 345 5977

BRITISH HOLISTIC MEDICAL ASSOCIATION
59 Lansdowne Place, Hove, East Sussex BN3 1FL
Tel/Fax: 01273 725951
Email: bhma@bhma.org

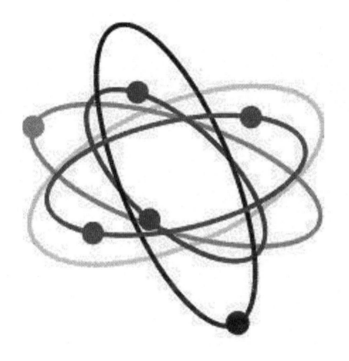

BRITISH INSTITUTE OF MAGNET THERAPY,
Lower Race, Pontypool, Torfaen NP4 5UH

BRITISH MEDICAL ACUPUNCTURE SOCIETY
Newton House, 12 Marbury House, Higher Whitley,
Warrington, Cheshire WA4 4QW
Tel: 01925 730727 Fax: 01925 730492
Email: admin@medical-acupuncture.org.uk

CONFEDERATION OF HEALING ORGANISATIONS
113 High Street, Northchurch, Berkhamsted,
Hertfordshire HP4 3QL
Tel: 01442 870667

NATIONAL OSTEOPOROSIS SOCIETY
Manor Farm, Skinners Hill, Camerton, Bath BA2 0PJ
Tel: 01761 471771